Psychiatric Symptoms and Comorbidities in Autism Spectrum Disorder

Luigi Mazzone • Benedetto Vitiello
Editors

Psychiatric Symptoms and Comorbidities in Autism Spectrum Disorder

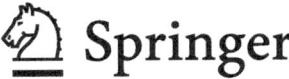 Springer

Editors
Luigi Mazzone
I.R.C.C.S. Bambino Gesù Children's Hospital
Rome
Italy

Benedetto Vitiello
National Institute of Mental Health
Bethesda, Maryland
USA

ISBN 978-3-319-29693-7   ISBN 978-3-319-29695-1   (eBook)
DOI 10.1007/978-3-319-29695-1

Library of Congress Control Number: 2016940095

Printed on acid-free paper

This Springer imprint is published by Springer Nature
The registered company is Springer International Publishing AG Switzerland

This book is dedicated to my love Lia, sweet woman and excellent researcher
(Luigi Mazzone)

Contents

Introduction

One of the most remarkable phenomena of the past twenty years has been the dramatic increase in the rate of the diagnosis of autism spectrum disorder (ASD) in our society. It is estimated that 1 in 68 children had been diagnosed with this disorder in 2010 in the USA (Department of Health and Human Services. Centers for Disease Control and Prevention, March 28, 2014).

This is a major increase over the 1 in 150 rate in 2000 and even the 1 in 88 rate in 2008. It is unclear how much of this phenomenon is accounted by the broader diagnostic criteria and the greater awareness for the condition among families, teachers, and clinicians, rather than by a true rise of the disorder (APA 2013). Regardless of the relative weight of the various possible causes, it is a fact that psychiatrists, pediatricians, neurologists, and primary care physicians are now much more likely to treat children with autism spectrum disorder in their daily practice than just a few years ago.

The management of autism spectrum disorder is typically complex and multidisciplinary. The core symptoms, consisting in deficits in social communication and language, and a pattern of restricted interests and repetitive behaviors, are best addressed with intensive psychoeducational programs that have been shown, on average, to ameliorate functioning (Dawson et al. 2010; Reichow et al. 2012). Treatment of associated medical problems, such as seizure disorders and gastrointestinal symptoms, is often needed. The management of behavioral problems in persons with autism spectrum disorder is an important challenge for clinicians and families, and the psychiatric symptoms in comorbidities could even exacerbate the behavioral dyscontrol.

Moreover, the symptoms of psychopathological conditions may be masked by those typical of ASD, and the threshold between autism spectrum core symptoms and comorbid symptoms can be blurred (Mazzone et al. 2012). Another common challenge for clinicians is to determine if psychiatric symptoms observed in ASD are part of the same dimension of autism spectrum itself or rather represent different categorical factors such as a psychiatric disorder in comorbidity. This happens because, as mentioned above, the core symptoms of ASD often mask the symptoms of the comorbid condition. A helpful strategy to disentangle this issue could be to look prospectively at the overall clinical outcome through longitudinal studies. Longitudinal studies allow researchers to closely follow the developmental trajectories of ASD and to detect subtle changes in behavior at different stages of development in terms of progressive appearance of clinical symptoms and impact of life experiences. Unfortunately, most of the clinical studies on ASD conducted so far typically have been cross-sectional, comparing one particular clinical measure at a single time point across samples. The interpretation of these cross-sectional findings is mostly focused on the abnormalities in the patient group as compared to healthy controls and on the contributions that these abnormal clinical abnormalities may have on disease evolution. If the need for longitudinal, prospective research is common to the study of all developmental psychopathology, it is especially crucial for ASD in order to understand the lifetime history of the disorder and the role of comorbid disorders. Indeed, children suffering from ASD have a different pattern of development compared to normal children, and their life experiences influence their cognitive and emotional status beginning within their first years of life.

An additional concern regards the suitability of the psychometric tools used in clinical practice to assess comorbid conditions in ASD. Of course, the psychiatric diagnosis of comorbidity relies on the competence of clinicians, but adequate tools such as scales or questionnaires adapted for ASD could be helpful to somehow standardize the recognition of psychiatric symptoms in this clinical sample. So far, most of the studies have used questionnaires, checklists, and scales designed for individuals with a normal awareness of their own and other's mental status. These instruments were not specifically adapted to take into account the neuropsychological characteristics of ASD in terms of deficits in mind reading, impairments in processing, and reporting their own feelings, emotions, and communication problems. Hence, new psychometric instruments, developed or adapted specifically to ASD, are needed.

These psychiatric symptoms substantially contribute to the burden of autism on patients and families. Even if not curative of the autism core deficits, successful management of associated psychiatric symptoms can lead to a significant improvement in functioning and quality of life (Arnold et al. 2003; Aman et al. 2009). Indeed the proper recognition and diagnosis of psychiatric comorbidities in ASD is also a crucial point for the pharmacological treatment of these individuals. The correct identification and attribution of overlapping symptoms either to the comorbid disorder or to the ASD itself may contribute to the choice of the most appropriate treatment for each one (Mazzone et al. 2012).

Psychiatric medications are commonly used in patients with autism spectrum disorder, with some studies showing use in up to one-third of children and two-thirds of adolescents (Coury et al. 2012). For years, this use has been based on anecdotal reports and expert opinion rather than on controlled investigations, thus raising concerns about both the efficacy and safety of these practices. More recently, research on the treatment of psychiatric symptoms in autism spectrum disorder has increased, and a number of controlled clinical trials have been conducted to test benefit and tolerability of several pharmacological and psychosocial interventions for the management of aggression, attention-deficit/hyperactivity disorder, and associated disruptive symptoms in children and adolescents with autism spectrum disorder (RUPP 2002; RUPP 2005; King et al. 2009; Scahill et al. 2015). This body of research data provides an evidence base for assessing the balance between potential benefits and risk, which is necessary for any rational use of interventions.

For example, we now know that certain agents, such as risperidone and aripiprazole, are highly effective in decreasing aggression and irritability, but their use can be accompanied by important metabolic adverse effects (Martin et al. 2004), or that methylphenidate is less effective and more likely to cause adverse effects when used for the management of ADHD in children with autism spectrum disorder as compared to ADHD without autism (RUPP 2005). And we also know that selective serotonin reuptake inhibitor medication is generally not effective in the management of repetitive behaviors in autism (King et al. 2009).

The integration of pharmacological treatment with psychosocial, educational, and rehabilitative interventions is a critical aspect of the management of autism spectrum disorder (Volkmar et al. 2014). Combining medication with behavioral intervention can be more effective in improving the level of functioning (Aman et al. 2009). As always in medicine, the treatment of the individual with autism spectrum disorder is an art that requires integration of the state-of-science data with the specific needs and characteristics of the patient. The purpose of this book is to provide clinicians with the most updated information on the diagnosis and treatment of common psychiatric symptoms associated with autism spectrum disorder, and it is meant to offer clinicians with the best scientific evidence on which to build successful therapeutic strategies for their patients.

The opinions and assertions here presented are the private views of the author, and are not to be construed as official statement of the National Institute of Mental Health, the National Institutes of Health, or the U.S. Department of Health and Human Services.

Rome, Italy   Luigi Mazzone
Bethesda, Maryland, USA   Benedetto Vitiello

References

1. Aman MG, McDougle CJ, Scahill L, Handen B, Arnold LE, Johnson C, Stigler KA, Karen Bearss K, Butter E, Swiezy NB, Sukhodolsky DD, Yaser Ramadan Y, Stacie L, Pozdol SL, Roumen Nikolov R, Lecavalier L, Arlene E. Kohn AE, Koenig K, Hollway JA, Korzekwa P, Gavaletz A, Mulick JA, Kristy L. Hall, Dziura J, Louise Ritz L, Trollinger S, Yu S, Vitiello B, Wagner A (2009) Medication and parent training in children with pervasive developmental disorders and serious behavior problems. J Am Acad Child Adolesc Psychiatry 48:1143–1154
2. American Psychiatric Association (2013) Diagnostic and Statistical Manual of Mental Disorders, 5th edn (DSM-5). American Psychiatric Association, Washington, DC
3. Arnold LE, Vitiello B, McDougle C, Scahill L, Shah B, Gonzalez NM, Chuang S, Davies M, Hollway J, Aman MG, Cronin P, Koenig K., Kohn AE, McMahon DJ, Tierney E (2003) Parent-defined target symptoms respond to risperidone in RUPP autism study: customer approach to clinical trials. J Am Acad Child Adolesc Psychiatry 42:1443–1450
4. Coury DL, Anagnostou E, Manning-Courtney P, Reynolds A, Cole L, McCoy R, Whitaker A, Perrin JM (2012) Use of psychotropic medication in children and adolescents with autism spectrum disorders. Pediatrics 130(Suppl 2):S69–S76

5. Dawson G, Rogers S, Munson J, Smith M, Winter J, Greenson J, Donaldson A, Varley J (2010) Randomized, controlled trial of an intervention for toddlers with autism: the Early Start Denver Model. Pediatrics 125(1):e17–23
6. King BH, Hollander E, Sikich L, McCracken JT, Scahill L, Bregman JD, Donnelly CL, Anagnostou E, Dukes K, Sullivan L, Hirtz D, Wagner A, Ritz L (2009) STAART Psychopharmacology Network. Lack of efficacy of citalopram in children with autism spectrum disorders and high levels of repetitive behavior: citalopram ineffective in children with autism. Arch Gen Psychiatry 66:583–590
7. Martin A, Scahill L, Anderson GM, Aman M, Arnold LE, McCracken J, McDougle CM, Tierney E, Chuang S, Vitiello B, and the Research Units on Pediatric Psychopharmaco-logy Autism Network (2004) Weight and leptin changes among risperidone-treated youths with autism: six-month prospective data. Am J Psychiatry 161:1125–1127
8. Mazzone L, Ruta L, Reale L (2012) Psychiatric comorbidities in asperger syndrome and high functioning autism: diagnostic challenges. Ann Gen Psychiatry 11:16
9. Reichow B, Barton EE, Boyd BA, Hume K (2012) Early intensive behavioral intervention (EIBI) for young children with autism spectrum disorders (ASD). Cochrane Database Syst Rev 10:CD009260.
10. Research Units on Pediatric Psychopharmacology Autism Network (2002) Risperidone in children with autism and serious behavioral problems. N Engl J Med 347:314–321
11. Research Units on Pediatric Psychopharmacology (RUPP) Autism Network (2005) A random-ized controlled crossover trial of methylphenidate in pervasive developmental disorders with hyperactivity. Arch Gen Psychiatry 62:1266–12174
12. Scahill L, McCracken JT, King BH, Rockhill C, Shah B, Politte L, Sanders R, Minjarez M, Cowen J, Mullett J, Page C, Ward D, Deng Y, Loo S, Dziura J, McDougle CJ (2015) Research Units on Pediatric Psychopharmacology Autism Network. Extended-release guanfacine for hyperactivity in children with autism spectrum disorder. Am J Psychiatry Aug 28:appi-ajp201515010055. [Epub ahead of print]
13. U.S. Department of Health and Human Services. Centers for Disease Control and Prevention. Prevalence of autism spectrum disorder among children aged 8 years—autism and develop-mental disabilities monitoring network, 11 Sites, United States, 2010. Morbidity and Mortality Weekly Report. Surveillance Summaries/Vol. 63/No. 2, 28 Mar 2014 (Available at Website http://www.cdc.gov/mmwr/pdf/ss/ss6302.pdf)
14. Volkmar F, Siegel M, Woodbury-Smith M, King B, McCracken J, State M, American Academy of Child and Adolescent Psychiatry (AACAP) Committee on Quality Issues (CQI) (2014) Practice parameter for the assessment and treatment of children and adolescents with autism spectrum disorder. J Am Acad Child Adolesc Psychiatry. 53:237–257

Mood Disorders and Autism Spectrum Disorder

Valentina Postorino, Stefano Vicari, and Luigi Mazzone

1 Introduction

Behavioral problems, which are often linked to psychiatric disorders in comorbidity in individuals with autism spectrum disorder (ASD), make the management of these patients even more difficult either for clinicians or families (Mazzone et al. 2012, 2013). Several studies documented high rates of psychiatric comorbidities in individuals with ASD, especially with regard to internalizing disorders. An association has been frequently reported with mood disorders, including depression and bipolar disorders (Hedley and Young 2006; Munesue et al. 2008; Simonoff et al. 2008, 2012). Internalizing symptoms are difficult to recognize in this clinical population because they can be misinterpret as features of autism. However, their identification represents a crucial point for both diagnosis and treatment (Mazzone et al. 2012, 2013). Therefore, understanding how mood symptoms (i.e., depression and mania) appear in individuals with ASD can help clinicians to delineate a correct distinction between these two conditions in order to develop adequate treatment strategies, either psychological or pharmacological. In this chapter we will describe the prevalence, the phenomenology and clinical features, the diagnostic process, neurobiological and genetic bases, and treatment of mood disorders in ASD.

V. Postorino (✉)
Department of Pediatrics, Marcus Autism Center, Emory University School of Medicine, Atlanta, GA, USA

Child Neuropsychiatry Unit, Department of Neuroscience, I.R.C.C.S. Bambino Gesù Children's Hospital, Rome, Italy
e-mail: valentina.postorino86@gmail.com

S. Vicari • L. Mazzone
Child Neuropsychiatry Unit, Department of Neuroscience, I.R.C.C.S. Bambino Gesù Children's Hospital, Rome, Italy
e-mail: stefano.vicari@opbg.net; luigi.mazzone@opbg.net

© Springer International Publishing Switzerland 2016
L. Mazzone, B. Vitiello (eds.), *Psychiatric Symptoms and Comorbidities in Autism Spectrum Disorder*, DOI 10.1007/978-3-319-29695-1_1

2   Prevalence

Studies published so far on the co-occurrence of ASD and mood disorders have reported variable prevalence rates ranging from 1.4 % to 70 % (Amr et al. 2012; Barnhill and Smith 2001; Brereton et al. 2006; Cassidy et al. 2014; De Bruin et al. 2007; Ghaziuddin and Greden 1998; Green et al. 2000; Gotham et al. 2014; Hedley and Young 2006; Henry et al. 2014; Hofvander et al. 2009; Joshi et al. 2013; Kim et al. 2000; Lainhart and Folstein 1994; Leyfer et al. 2006; Lugnegård et al. 2011; Mazefsky et al. 2011; Mazzone et al. 2013; Mattila et al. 2010; Munesue et al. 2008; Pouw et al. 2013; Rosenberg et al. 2011; Simonoff et al. 2008, 2012; Stahlberg et al. 2004; Sterling et al. 2008; Strang et al. 2012; Vickerstaff et al. 2007; Whitehouse et al. 2009; Williamson et al. 2008; Wozniak et al. 1997). However, all these studies used different diagnostic criteria, reasons for referral, and age ranges; thus these issues could account for these wide rates. Indeed, these discrepancies could be explained by the level of intellectual ability of the patients enrolled. In fact, studies involving individuals with ASD and intellectual disability (ID) generally report slightly lower rate of co-occurring mood disorders in this population (De Bruin et al. 2007; Hofvander et al. 2009; Rosenberg et al. 2011). For instance, De Bruin et al. (2007) in a sample of 94 children with Pervasive Developmental Disorder-Not Otherwise Specified (PDD-NOS) reported that 13.8 % of them had at least one mood disorder of which major depression occurred most frequently (10.6 %). However, patients enrolled in this study reported a highly variable intellectual ability (intelligence quotient (IQ) ranging from 55 to 120). Similarly, a recent study examining variation in cumulative prevalence of community diagnosis of psychiatric comorbidity in 4,343 children with ASD, and including 1,170 individuals with an ID, found that 11 % of them showed a comorbid depression and 5.2 % a bipolar disorder (Rosenberg et al. 2011). On the other hand, individuals with high-functioning autism (HFA) seem to be particularly affected by mood disorders (Ghaziuddin and Greden 1998; Kim et al. 2000; Mazzone et al. 2013; Munesue et al. 2008; Stewart et al. 2006; Vickerstaff et al. 2007; Whitehouse et al. 2009). For instance, two recent studies investigating depressive symptoms in HFA samples through self-report questionnaires found that these patients reported severe depressive symptoms (Mazzone et al. 2013; Whitehouse et al. 2009). Moreover, Ghaziuddin and Greden (1998) reported a rate of mood disorders of 34 % in a sample of 35 patients with a diagnosis of Asperger Syndrome (AS). In line with these results, a recent study found that 16 out of 44 outpatients with HFA (36.4 %) had a comorbid mood disorder (Munesue et al. 2008). Higher rates of co-occurrence of bipolar I disorder and ASD were obtained in a large controlled analysis of phenotypic and familiar correlates in a referred population of youth with bipolar I disorder assessed for the comorbidity with ASD (Joshi et al. 2013). Specifically, these authors reported that 30.3 % of the bipolar I probands met criteria for ASD (Joshi et al. 2013). Generally, in adolescent and adult patients with HFA, the rates of comorbid mood disorders seem to be even higher (Cassidy et al. 2014; Hofvander et al. 2009; Lugnegård et al. 2011; Stahlberg et al. 2004; Sterling et al. 2008). In more detail, Hofvander et al. (2009) reported that the most common lifetime comorbid condition was mood disorders (53 %) in a sample of adolescents and adults with ASD without ID. Moreover, Lugnegård et al. (2011) investigating psychiatric comorbidity in young adults with a clinical diagnosis of AS reported that 70 % of adults with ASD had experienced at least one major episode of depression and 50 % of them had suffered from recurrent depressive episodes. Indeed, a recent clinical cohort study on 374 adults with AS found that 32 % of the sample reported a history of depression (Cassidy et al. 2014).

3   Phenomenology and Clinical Issues

Autistic symptoms can mask psychiatric disorders in comorbidity, and thereby shedding light on the phenomenology of mood symptoms in ASD is a clinical issue (Frazier et al. 2002; Lainhart and Folstein 1994; Magnuson and Constantino 2011; Mazzone et al. 2012, 2013, 2014; Simonoff et al. 2008). Depressive symptoms (e.g., social withdrawal and blunt affect) can be easily covered by some of the core autistic symptoms if not specifically investigated. During the diagnostic process, clinicians have to keep in mind that the clinical manifestation of depressive symptoms in patients with ASD may involve generic depressive clinical signs (e.g., increase in crying, self-injury, decrease in activity with a loss of interest in the daily living, apathy, anhedonia, feelings of guilt, low self-esteem, and recurrent thought of death) (Ghaziuddin et al. 2002; Mazzone et al. 2012; Vannucchi et al. 2014). Furthermore, as in other patients with depressive symptoms, the neurovegetative symptoms can be present (e.g., changes in appetite and weight or sleep disturbance, including hypersomnia, insomnia, or reversal of day and night). On the other hand, there are some possible depressive symptoms which could be more specific in ASD. These might include irritability, a change in repetitive and stereotyped behavior, or an increase in compulsive behaviors (Ghaziuddin et al. 2002; Gotham et al. 2014). For instance, clinicians has to consider that a temporary decrease of repetitive and stereotyped behaviors in individuals with ASD can be either an improvement of autistic symptoms or a manifestation of depressive symptoms (Lainhart and Folstein 1994; O'Brien et al. 2001; Stewart et al. 2006; Tantam 2000; Weissman and Bates 2010; Wing 1996). Age of onset of a co-occurring depression is predominantly around pre-adolescence and adolescence, probably because during this period of transition these patients become more aware of their own social skills (Ghaziuddin et al. 2002; Mazzone et al. 2012; Williamson et al. 2008). Indeed, several studies suggest that the rate of depression in individuals with ASD increases with age, as well as the lower self-perceived social competence (Brereton et al. 2006; Ghaziuddin et al. 2002; Vickerstaff et al. 2007). Another clinical symptom of depression peculiar of individuals with ASD is the regression often observed in this clinical population during lifespan. It is particularly observed in individuals with low functioning autism and might be characterized by loss of language, social withdrawal, loss of eye contact, moodiness, tantrums, fearfulness, obsessiveness, stereotypies, hyperactivity, and occasionally self-injurious behaviors (Ghaziuddin et al. 2002; Myers and Winters 2002).

Other factors that can play an important role in the onset of mood disorders in ASD are environmental factors: stressors and negative life events (i.e., family sickness, change of house, or bereavement) may contribute to the occurrence of depression in individuals with ASD (Ghaziuddin et al. 1995). It is well known that patients with depression have experience of increasing stressors before illness onset (Brown and Harris 1989; Hammen 2005). Therefore, the experience of these negative life events could play a role in the occurrence of this disorder also in people with autism. According to this, Ghaziuddin et al. (1995) have investigated the presence of independent negative life events in two groups of children with pervasive developmental disorder (PDD) (11 patients with PDD and 11 patients with PDD and depression) for a period of 12 months prior to onset of depression. Findings indicated that 82 % of children with PDD and a comorbid depression had a history of recent unpleasant life events as compared to 45 % of the group with PDD without depression.

Regarding bipolar disorders the symptoms that could strongly suggest their occurrence in individuals with autism are manic and hypomanic signs (e.g., irritable, instable and dysphoric mood, excessive reactivity, hyperarousal, agitation, flight of ideas, pressured speech, increase distractibility, poor judgment, intrusiveness, laughing, aggression, and noncompliance) (Lainhart and Folstein 1994; Joshi et al. 2013; Skeppar et al. 2013; Vannucchi et al. 2014). In clinical practice it is common to misinterpret affective signs as features of schizophrenia in patients with ASD (Skeppar et al. 2013). Generally, it has to be considered that bizarre thoughts are different from odd thinking and stereotypic ideas and feelings which are common in this clinical population. Even though in individuals with ASD these bizarre ideas may become more pronounced and intense during manic episodes, these are stable and preexisting since childhood (Vannucchi et al. 2014).

In order to make a correct distinction between these conditions, clinicians has to consider that manic symptoms in autism (e.g., hyperarousal or excessive reactivity) may simply be caused by impairments in social understanding, instead of being clinical signs of co-occurring mood disorders (Mazzone et al. 2012). A recent study has investigated the phenotypic and familial correlates of bipolar disorder when it occurs with and without ASD in order to understand if these correlates of bipolar disorder could be comparable despite the comorbidity with autism (Joshi et al. 2013). Results revealed that the phenotypic features of bipolar disorder were similar in youth with and without ASD comorbidity, with an age of onset of bipolar disorder significantly earlier when there was a comorbidity with autism (Joshi et al. 2013). Thus, this study suggested that the phenotypic and familial correlates are typical and specific of the bipolar disorder despite the presence of ASD comorbidity. Similarly, Wozniak et al. (1997) investigating the overlap between mania and PDD in a consecutive sample of referred youths found that 21 % of these children reported both disorders. Moreover, supporting the independence of the two syndromes, the autistic symptoms were identical in children with autism irrespective of the comorbidity with mania (Wozniak et al. 1997). In addition, the clinical features and the course of mania, such as irritable mood and chronic course, were similar in manic children with and without autism (Wozniak et al. 1997). These results provide preliminary evidence of a peculiar clinical profile in children with both conditions. However, further studies better characterizing the different clinical and neurocognitive impairments experienced by youth with ASD with and without bipolar disorder are needed in order to shed light on the different clinical characteristics of these conditions and help clinicians in the diagnostic process.

4 Peculiar Features of Mood Disorders in ASD

4.1 Relation Between Cognitive Ability and Mood Symptoms in Patients with ASD

Cognitive ability is a factor that seems to account the occurrence of a mood disorder in autism. HFA are more likely to develop mood symptoms (Cassidy et al. 2014; Ghaziuddin et al. 2002; Ghaziuddin and Greden 1998; Hofvander et al. 2009; Kim et al. 2000; Lugnegård et al. 2011; Mazzone et al. 2013; Munesue et al. 2008; Stahlberg et al. 2004; Sterling et al. 2008; Stewart et al. 2006; Vickerstaff et al. 2007; Whitehouse et al. 2009). A factor that can contribute to this higher rate is that even if these individuals could be interested in social interaction, they may not have the appropriate skills to successfully develop social relationships (Barnhill and Smith 2001). Generally they report difficulties in social functioning, including make friends and maintain peer relationship, thus experiencing loneliness (Brunstein Klomek et al. 2007; Little 2002; Humphrey and Lewis 2008; Mazurek 2014; Whitehouse et al. 2009). A recent study on the relationship between social functioning and depressive symptoms in children with HFA compared to a group of typically developing children reported that the former showed more maladaptive coping strategies and poorer social functioning which were uniquely associated with more symptoms of depression (Pouw et al. 2013). Therefore, a person with ASD and an average or above-average cognitive ability probably experiences multiple failures in different social contests (e.g., school, family, etc.). The experience of these social failures can lead to a lower self-esteem, which, in turn, increases the risk for depression (Ozonoff et al. 2002).

A possible explanation of the lower occurrence of depression in individuals with autism and ID is that the abilities to process and perceive these social failures as negative experiences could be compromised in this clinical population; thereby the risk to develop depressive symptoms is decreased.

Another possible hypothesis for the higher association of depressive symptoms in HFA is that these individuals can misinterpret social situation since they are not able to make inferences regarding own and others' state of mind. These difficulties seem to be particularly pronounced during adolescence, a developmental period in which the social identification becomes essential (Simonoff et al. 2008; Sterling et al. 2008). For instance, Strang et al. (2012) examining the relationship between age, IQ, autism, and depressive symptoms in school-age children and adolescents with ASD and an average IQ, through a parent-report questionnaire that investigates behavioral problems (i.e., Child Behavior Checklist (CBCL)), reported that 30 % of the sample was in the clinical range for depression.

4.2   Co-occurrence of Catatonia as an Exacerbation of Mood Symptoms in ASD

Catatonia is a disorder of movement that can occur in the context of several psychiatric disorders and other medical conditions (American Psychiatric Association 2013). In the Diagnostic and Statistical Manual-5th edition (DSM-5), catatonia is defined by the presence of 3 or more of 12 psychomotor features and is not considered as an independent disorder, but as a specifier for a mental disorder (i.e., neurodevelopmental disorder, psychotic disorder, depressive disorder, bipolar disorder, or other mental disorders) or due to another medical condition (APA 2013). Currently, literature studies suggest an increased recognition of catatonia as a comorbid disorder of ASD (Billstedt et al. 2005; Fink et al. 2006; Fink and Taylor 2003; Mazzone et al. 2014; Takaoka and Takata 2007; Wing and Shah 2000). However, given the overlap of symptoms between these conditions, such as mutism, stereotypic speech, repetitive behaviors, echolalia, posturing, mannerisms, purposeless agitation, and rigidity, in clinical practice it is difficult to make a correct distinction between catatonia and ASD (Dhossche et al. 2006; Dhossche 2004; Mazzone et al. 2014). The broad clinical presentation of catatonia symptoms, ranging from marked unresponsiveness to marked agitation, leads the recognition of this comorbidity in ASD even more challenging. Generally, it should be taken into account that catatonia appears at a later age than autistic symptoms, and an assessment of a comorbid catatonia in patients with autism should be considered only if a change in type and pattern of preexisting symptoms is observed (Mazzone et al. 2013; Wing and Shah 2000). Although historically catatonia has been linked to schizophrenia, recent studies have highlighted that in the majority of cases this syndrome involves individual with mood disorders (i.e., depression and bipolar disorders) (Fink 2013; Fink et al. 2006; Fink and Taylor 2003). Therefore, as in this clinical population, even in patients with autism, catatonia could be an exacerbation of mood symptoms already present (Mazzone et al. 2014). For instance, Fink et al. (2006) in a series of six case reports with a history of autism and a comorbid catatonia suggested that catatonia in patients with ASD can be thought of as the comorbidity with a mood disorder instead of a separate disorder. Moreover, given that mood symptoms are difficult to recognize in patients with ASD, the marked clinical presentation of catatonic presentation is sometimes an easier and only way to identify previous mood alteration already present in this clinical population.

5   Diagnosis and Evaluation: Assessment Tools

The assessment of mood symptoms in this clinical population is particularly complex because of the reduced ability of these patients for introspection and problems in communicating their personal state (Ghaziuddin et al. 2002; Lainhart 1999). Regarding this last point, the recognition of comorbid mood disorders in individuals with ASD and ID is even more difficult because in this clinical population the impairment of these abilities might be even higher. Currently, to our knowledge, only four tools were specifically developed to assess comorbid psychopathology in autism and tested in this clinical population: (1) Autism Comorbidity Interview-Present and Lifetime Version (ACI-PL), a modification of the Kiddie-Schedule for Affective Disorders and Schizophrenia-Present and Lifetime Version (K-SADS-PL) to make it more appropriate for use in autism; (2) the Autism Spectrum Disorders-Comorbidity for Children (ASD-CC), a 49-item rating scale designed to assess symptoms of emotional difficulties which commonly occur in children with ASD; (3) the Autism Spectrum Disorders-Comorbidity for Adults (ASD-CA), 84-item scale designed to look at comorbid psychopathology in adults with ASD and ID; and (4) the Psychopathology in Autism Checklist (PAC), a checklist discriminating between autism and four major psychiatric disorders (i.e., psychosis, depression, anxiety, and obsessive-compulsive disorder) (Helverschou et al. 2009; Kaufman et al. 1997; Leyfer et al. 2006; Matson et al. 2009, Matson and Wilkins 2008; Matson and Boisjoli 2003; Thorson and Matson 2012). However, these instruments investigate psychiatric comorbidities in general, and to date diagnostic tools specifically created and validated to investigate the presence of mood disorders in patients with ASD are still lacking. In fact, the instruments usually used are structured or semi-structured clinical interviews based on the DSM criteria, which investigate multiple domains of psychopathology, including mood symptoms (Kaufman et al. 1997; Mazzone et al. 2012, 2013; Shaffer et al. 2000; Spitzer et al. 1994; Welner et al. 1987). Furthermore, these diagnostic tools have been designed and standardized referring to the general population and as such likely not appropriate for ASD (Mazzone et al. 2012, 2013). Parent-report questionnaires are also often used, but these instruments only inquire about current symptoms (Achenbach 1991; Gracious et al. 2002). Self-report questionnaires have been widely used (Allgaier et al. 2014; Beck et al. 1961; Brink et al. 1982; Esbensen et al. 2003; Frühe et al. 2012; Hamilton 1960; Kovacs 1982; Radloff 1977; Young et al. 1978; Zigmond and Snaith 1983). However, many items of these scales require metacognitive abilities (e.g., such as awareness, self-awareness, and auto-consciousness) which may be problematic for patients with ASD. Therefore, this issue makes these tools not appropriate for this clinical population. For instance, the Children's Depression Inventory (CDI) is a self-report scale in which the child or the adolescent has to choose among three options indicating increasing severity of depressive symptoms, including the presence of negative mood, interpersonal difficulties, negative self-esteem, and ineffectiveness (Kovacs 1982). Noticeable is that, in order to rate the presence of these symptoms, the abilities to understand and report own and others' feeling and emotions should be unimpaired. However, even in presence of average language and cognitive skills, autistic patients might have a deficit in these competencies. Indeed, even clinician-rated instruments, such as the Children's Depression Rating Scale-Revised (CDRS-R), a 17-item clinical interview for child, parent, and teacher investigating the severity of depressive symptoms, require intact metacognitive skills, including the ability to describe their mental states, mental experiences, and daily life experiences (Leyfer et al. 2006; Poznanski and Mokros 1996). Hence, this issue affects the sensitivity of these instruments (Mazzone et al. 2012).

In fact, literature studies report a lack of correspondence between self-report screeners and parent-reported psychiatric diagnosis that could be explained by the metacognitive difficulties of autistic patients (Mazefsky et al. 2011).

In order to reduce the discrepancy created by these diagnostic issues, it is recommended a deep evaluation of the history and development. Moreover, it is fundamental that the clinician gathers information from multiple sources (e.g., patents, parents, teachers, etc.) and settings in order to have a complete picture of the patient and distinguish between these conditions (Jepsen et al. 2012; Magnuson and Constantino 2011; Mazzone et al. 2012, 2013).

6 Neurobiological Bases for the Relation Between ASD and Mood Disorders

Shedding light on the neurobiological bases and defining the mechanisms underlying autism and mood disorders is a crucial issue in order to delineate the distinct features of these conditions. Analyzing the neurobiological systems can contribute to illustrate which are the relations between these disorders. Even though abnormalities in brain functioning and structures have been described either in autistic or mood disorder patients, to our knowledge only one study compared brain structures (i.e., caudate volume) in these clinical populations (Kerestes et al. 2013; Mazzone and Curatolo 2010; Voelbel et al. 2006; Wiggins et al. 2012; Zhang et al. 2014). Therefore, we decided to focus this section on the genetic and biological basis of these disorders.

6.1 Genetic Overlap Between ASD and Mood Disorders

A growing body of evidences supports that both ASD and mood disorders are high heritable genetic pathologies. Broad rates of association between these disorders suggest that their genetic and biological basis could be partially shared or that a common etiological pathway may exist (Magnuson and Constantino 2011; Munesue et al. 2008; Ragunath et al. 2011; Scherff et al. 2014). However, to date, little is known about the causes of the occurrence of mood disorders in autism. Several researches have tried to clarify the relationship between ASD and mood disorders, but only a few studies assessed the etiological factors associated between these disorders within a genetic model and the available findings have shown contrasting results (Ghaziuddin et al. 2002; Mazzone et al. 2012, 2013; Ragunath et al. 2011). A recent study has identified common pathways and genes involved in ASD and bipolar disorder using independently two different tools: consensus path database (a molecular functional interaction database that integrates information from different manually curated pathway on protein interaction, metabolism, genetic interaction signaling, and gene regulation) and GeneGO pathway maps (an integrated functional software suite for functional analysis of genetic data) were employed for the analysis (Kamburov et al. 2009; Ragunath et al. 2011). These tools identified four pathways common to both disorders: the synaptic transmission pathway, the neuroactive ligand receptor interaction pathway, the circadian rhythm pathway, and the catecholamine biosynthesis pathway. All these pathways are involved in several functions, such as regulating stress or maintaining mood, implicated in both ASD and bipolar disorder. Therefore, it has been suggested that the comorbidity of these disorders can be correlated to the genes involved in the pathways shared by the two disorders (Ragunath et al. 2011). Moreover, a recent genome-wide analysis for five psychiatric disorders (i.e., ASD, major depressive disorder, bipolar disorder, attention deficit-hyperactivity disorder (ADHD), and schizophrenia) conducted by the Psychiatric Genomics Consortium with the aim of identifying specific variants underlying genetic effects shared between these disorders showed a reduced, but still significant, overlap between aggregate genetic risk for ASD with schizophrenia and bipolar disorder (Cross-Disorder Group of the Psychiatric Genomics Consortium 2013a). However, no significant polygenetic overlap was detected between ASD and major depressive disorder or ADHD. On the other hand, another study performed by the same research group and examining the genetic relationship between these five psychiatric disorders estimated from genome-wide single-nucleotide polymorphisms (SNPs) reported a low genetic correlation between ASD and schizophrenia but nonsignificant correlations for ASD and the other three disorders (Cross-Disorder Group of the Psychiatric Genomics Consortium 2013b). Nonetheless, as stated by the authors of this study, it should be pointed out that the sample sizes varied widely across the five psychiatric disorders; thus the nonsignificant associations could reflect a lack power to detect common associated variants of small effect instead of the actual absence of this association.

Indeed, some studies have hypothesized a bidirectional influence between autistic-like traits and internalizing symptoms (Hallett et al. 2010, 2012; Pine et al. 2008; Scherff et al. 2014; Towbin et al. 2005). For instance, Hallett et al. (2012) in a community-based twin study investigated both phenotypic and etiological associations between autistic-like traits and internalizing traits, in 7.311 twin pairs aged 7 and 8 years. Results showed a phenotypic correlation and a genetic association between autistic-like traits (i.e., social difficulties, communication problems, and repetitive/restricted behaviors) and internalizing traits (i.e., social anxiety, fears, generalized anxiety, and negative affect). Considering that the majority of studies suggest a genetic overlap between ASD and mood disorders, but the available findings are still unclear, further researches are needed in order to identify specific genes that can contribute to comorbidity. Shedding light on this issue could help to develop novel management strategies and therapeutics techniques.

6.2   The Role of Serotonin in Autism and Mood Disorders

A pivotal role in the relationship between autism and mood disorders could be played by serotonin (5-HT). This neurotransmitter influences many functions in the central nervous system (CNS) and periphery system (e.g., regulating mood, sleep, food intake, body temperature, arousal, moderating pain sensitivity, sleep, aggression, affective, sexual behavior, and hormone release) and, during early stages, plays an important role in brain development (Chugani 2002; Meyer 2013). Research studies have reported that 5-HT is involved in the development of psychiatric disorders, and in many of these disorders, including autism, depression, and bipolar disorders, a dysregulation of the serotoninergic system has been described (Blier and El Mansari 2013; Chugani 2002; Jiang et al. 2013; Kepser and Homberg 2015). The role of the 5-HT system in the development of major depressive disorder has been widely described through the studies on the therapeutic efficacy of antidepressant treatments (Blier and El Mansari 2013). However, only little is known about the mechanism underlying autism. Hyperserotonemia, that is, the increase of 5-HT in blood, is generally the most widely described change in individuals with autism, observed in one third of this clinical population (Cook and Leventhal 1996; Coutinho et al. 2007; Janusonis 2005; Kepser and Homberg 2015; Meyer 2013; Ramoz et al. 2006; Veenstra-vanderweele et al. 2001). A recent review investigating the potential causes of ASD suggests that elevated cortisol levels during pregnancy increase the expression of the serotonin reuptake transporter (SERT), consequently altering the serotonin levels during gestation and modifying prenatal neuronal development in children with ASD. Prenatal conditions that elevate cortisol levels, thus increasing the risk for ASD, include hypertension, gestational diabetes, and depression (Meyer 2013). Thus, a possible prevention for autism could be the establishment of a standard protocol to measure cortisol levels during pregnancy. Indeed, given that depression can negatively influence the neurodevelopment of unborns and newborns, treatment of this disorder is crucial. Selective serotonin reuptake inhibitors (SSRIs) are the most frequently prescribed medication for the treatment of depression, even for depressed pregnant and postpartum women (Nonacs and Cohen 2003). Nonetheless, SSRIs increase 5-HT levels by inhibiting its reuptake, and prenatal and postnatal SSRI exposures are indicated as risk factors for autism. For this reason non-drug treatments, such as cognitive-behavioral therapy (CBT), could be a possible strategy in order to prevent the risk of newborn affected by autism (Cuijpers et al. 2013; Strauss et al. 2014). Consequently, further studies on the efficacy of these treatments in depressed pregnant women are essential in order to help clinicians to choose the optimal treatment. Finally, a recent study supporting the important role of 5-HT in human affect and sociality in disorders like depression and autism proposed an interaction between 5-HT and oxytocin (OXT) in areas of the brain important for the regulation of emotion-based behaviors (Mottolese et al. 2014). Specifically, these authors highlighted the role of OXT in the inhibitory regulation of 5-HT signaling, thus suggesting that these neuromodulators should be considered in order to implement novel therapeutic strategies for these disorders.

7   Treatments

7.1   Non-medical Treatments

Some evidence is reported on the psychotherapy treatments for mood disorders in ASD. Non-medical treatments for mood symptoms in autism have been focused on the application of CBT interventions, implemented through individual- or group-based settings (Brosnan and Healy 2011; Cardaciotto and Herbert 2004; Dawson and Burner 2011; Kuroda et al. 2013; Reichow et al. 2012; Sofronoff et al. 2007; Weiss and Lunsky 2010). However, its efficacy in treating depressive symptoms in autistic individuals has only been studied to a limited extent.

The majority of interventions have been developed for the treatment of associated symptoms in individual with autism (i.e., aggression, impaired social skills, theory of mind, or the improvement of emotion recognition and regulation) thus not focused on mood symptoms (Brosnan and Healy 2011; Cardaciotto and Herbert 2004; Dawson and Burner 2011; Kuroda et al. 2013; Reichow et al. 2012; Sofronoff et al. 2007). For instance, Kuroda et al. (2013) in a randomized control trial (RCT) of CBT for emotion regulation in adults with ASD examined 60 adults with autism and demonstrated the efficacy of CBT for improving the ability of these patients to identify their own and others' mental states. In line with these results, Sofronoff et al. (2007) in a RCT on anger management in children with AS revealed the efficacy of a small group CBT intervention to help children with autism with anger control. Notice that recent researches have also described limitation of this therapy for this clinical population. In fact, cognitive restructuring, which is one of the techniques used in CBT interventions, is useful for understanding unhappy feelings and moods and for challenging the sometimes-wrong "automatic beliefs" that can lie behind them. However, the concept of cognitive restructuring could be very difficult to learn for individuals with autism for their impairment in understand their own mental states. Moreover, generalization to real-life situations of cognitive-behavioral techniques is arduous. Mindfulness-based therapy (MBT) may also prove to be a useful therapeutic technique to reduce depression in ASD populations (Hofmann et al. 2010; Spek et al. 2013; Teasdale et al. 1995). Mindfulness has been defined as paying attention to experiences in the present moment in a nonjudgmental and accepting way, and its efficacy has been proved in treating patients with mood disorders (Hofmann et al. 2010; Kabat-Zinn 1990; Teasdale et al. 1995). This method encourages individuals to identify feelings or thoughts in the present moment and accept them, as they appear without analysis or discussion, an approach that may be well suited to those with theory of mind and communication deficits. Recently, Spek et al. (2013) carried out a first RCT aimed at investigating the beneficial effect of a MBT intervention in adults with ASD in treating comorbid affective symptoms. The results of this study showed a reduction in depression and rumination and an increase in positive affect in the intervention group as opposed to the control group, thus supporting the importance to examine this technique in the treatment of comorbid depression in patients with ASD.

7.2 Pharmacological Interventions

Data on the pharmacological intervention in individuals with ASD and comorbid mood disorders is scarce and consists only of case reports and open-label trials (RCTs are lacking) (Frazier et al. 2002; Joshi et al. 2012; King 2000; Siegel et al.

2014; Vannucchi et al. 2014). Moreover, the majority of these studies have investigated the effectiveness and tolerability of pharmacological treatments in treating target symptoms frequently associated with autism and highly suggestive of a comorbid mood disorder (i.e., irritability, self-injurious behaviors, severe tantrum, and aggression) (Hellings et al. 2005; Hollander et al. 2010; Kimberly 2014; Kirino 2014). Currently, risperidone and aripiprazole are the only two medications approved for these symptoms in autism (Findling et al. 2014; Marcus et al. 2009; McDougle et al. 1997; Kimberly 2014; Politte et al. 2014; Stachnik and Nunn-Thompson 2007). Regarding the effectiveness of other second-generation antipsychotics (SGA) (i.e., quetiapine, olanzapine, and ziprasidone) for the treatment of irritability associated with autism, the studies report inconsistent results (Kimberly 2014; Politte et al. 2014).

Lithium has been widely used as a mood stabilizer in autistic individuals, and studies have supported the efficacy of this drug, especially, for manic symptoms (Epperson et al. 1994; Frazier et al. 2002; Siegel et al. 2014). However, it has to be noticed that the available findings on lithium in this clinical population are based only on the limited literature data reported in case reports and case series. Furthermore, among the mood-stabilizing anticonvulsants, the effects of divalproex sodium have been widely examined and it has been suggested the efficacy of this medication for the treatment of irritability and aggression in patients with autism (Hollander et al. 2010; Kimberly 2014). Concerning tricyclic antidepressant (TCA) and SSRI for treating depression in patients with ASD, the evidences are limited and conflicting (Hurwitz et al. 2012; Vannucchi et al. 2014). Generally, when these treatment options are used, the clinicians should be aware of their relevant side effects, such as an increment of hyperactivity, aggression, and suicidal thoughts, especially in children and adolescents, and a continuous monitoring of these medications is recommended.

Summarizing, when a patient with ASD and a comorbid mood disorder is unresponsive or insufficiently responsive to non-medical treatments, a pharmacological interventions can be explored. However, caution is warranted given that RCTs on medication in this clinical population are lacking, and further research is needed on this topic.

8   Discussion and Future Directions

Further studies are needed on the prevalence rate of the co-occurrence of these disorders. Indeed, shedding light on the phenomenology of mood symptoms in this clinical population is a crucial issue given that the presence of comorbid disorders seems to be a negative prognostic factor on outcome of patients with ASD (Fein et al. 2013; Orinstein et al. 2014; Troyb et al. 2014). Indeed, the need of proper screening tools specifically designed for this population and the study of the mechanisms underlying these disorders have been described. Finally, given the lack of RCT on medical and psychological treatments, longitudinal controlled studies are essential in order to provide evidence-based guidelines for clinicians and therapists.

References

Achenbach TM (1991) Child behavior checklist. Psychological Corporation, San Antonio

Allgaier AK, Krick K, Opitz A, Saravo B, Romanos M, Schulte-Körne G (2014) Improving early detection of childhood depression in mental health care: the children's depression screener (ChilD-S). Psychiatry Res 217(3):248–252

American Psychiatric Association (2013) Diagnostic and statistical manual of mental disorders, 5th edn. American Psychiatric Association, Washington, DC

Amr M, Raddad D, El-Mehesh F, Bakr A, Sallam K, Amin T (2012) Comorbid psychiatric disorders in Arab children with autism spectrum disorders. Res Aut Spectrum Disord 6:240–248

Barnhill GP, Smith MB (2001) Attributional style and depression in adolescents with Asperger syndrome. J Posit Behav Interv 3:175–182

Beck AT, Ward CH, Mendelson M, Mock J, Erbaugh J (1961) An inventory for measuring depression. Arch Gen Psychiatry 4:561–571

Billstedt E, Gilberg C, Gilberg C (2005) Autism after adolescence: population-based 13- to 22-year follow-up study of 120 individuals with autism diagnosed in childhood. J Autism Dev Disord 35:351–360

Blier P, El Mansari M (2013) Serotonin and beyond: therapeutics for major depression. Philos Trans R Soc Lond B Biol Sci 25(1615):368

Brereton AV, Tonge BJ, Einfeld SL (2006) Psychopathology in children and adolescents with autism compared to young people with intellectual disability. J Autism Dev Disord 36(7):863–870

Brink TL, Yesavage JA, Lum O, Heersema PH, Adey M, Rose TL (1982) Screening tests for geriatric depression. Clin Gerontol 1:37–43

Brosnan J, Healy O (2011) A review of behavioral interventions for the treatment of aggression in individuals with developmental disabilities. Res Dev Disabil 32:437–446

Brown GW, Harris TO (1989) Life events and illness. Guilford, New York

Brunstein Klomek A, Marrocco F, Kleinman M, Schonfeld IS, Gould MS (2007) Bullying, depression, and suicidality in adolescents. J Am Acad Child Adolesc Psychiatry 46(1):40–49

Cardaciotto L, Herbert JD (2004) Cognitive behavior therapy for social anxiety disorder in the context of Asperger's syndrome: a single-subject report. Cogn Behav Pract 11:75–81

Cassidy S, Bradley P, Robinson J, Allison C, McHugh M, Baron-Cohen S (2014) Suicidal ideation and suicide plans or attempts in adults with Asperger's syndrome attending a specialist diagnostic clinic: a clinical cohort study. Lancet Psychiatry 1:142–147

Chugani DC (2002) Role of altered brain serotonin mechanisms in autism. Mol Psychiatry 7(Suppl 2):S16–S17

Cook EH, Leventhal BL (1996) The serotonin system in autism. Curr Opin Pediatr 8(4):348–354

Coutinho AM, Sousa I, Martins M, Correia C, Morgadinho T, Bento C, Marques C, Ataíde A, Miguel TS, Moore JH, Oliveira G, Vicente AM (2007) Evidence for epistasis between SLC6A4 and ITGB3 in autism etiology and in the determination of platelet serotonin levels. Hum Genet 121(2):243–256

Cross-Disorder Group of the Psychiatric Genomics Consortium (2013a) Identification of risk loci with shared effects on five major psychiatric disorders: a genome-wide analysis. Lancet 381:1371–1379

Cross-Disorder Group of the Psychiatric Genomics Consortium (2013b) Genetic relationship between five psychiatric disorders estimated from genome-wide SNPs. Nat Genet 45(9):984–994

Cuijpers P, Berking M, Andersson G, Quigley L, Kleiboer A, Dobson KS (2013) A meta-analysis of cognitive-behavioural therapy for adult depression, alone and in comparison with other treatments. Can J Psychiatry 58(7):376–385

Dawson G, Burner K (2011) Behavioral interventions in children and adolescents with autism spectrum disorder: a review of recent findings. Curr Opin Pediatr 23:616–620

De Bruin EI, Ferdinand RF, Meester S, de Nijs PF, Verheij F (2007) High rates of psychiatric co-morbidity in PDD-NOS. J Autism Dev Disord 37(5):877–886

Dhossche DM (2004) Autism as early expression of catatonia. Med Sci Monit 10(3):RA 31–RA 39

Dhossche D, Shah A, Wing L (2006) Blueprints for the assessment, treatment, and future study of catatonia in autism spectrum disorders. Int Rev Neurobiol 72:267–284

Epperson CN, McDougle CJ, Anand A, Marek GJ, Naylor ST, Volkmar FR, Donald JC, Lawrence HP (1994) Lithium augmentation of fluvoxamine in autistic disorder: a case report. J Child Adolesc Psychopharmacol 4(3):201–207

Esbensen AJ, Rojahn J, Aman MJ, Ruedrich S (2003) Reliability and validity of an assessment instrument for anxiety, depression, and mood among individuals with mental retardation. J Autism Dev Disord 33(6):617–629

Fein D, Barton M, Eigsti IM, Kelley E, Naigles L, Schultz RT, Stevens M, Helt M, Orinstein A, Rosenthal M, Troyb E, Tyson K (2013) Optimal outcome in individuals with a history of autism. Child Psychol Psychiatry 54(2):195–205

Findling R, Mankoski R, Timko K, Lears K, McCartney T, McQuade RD, Eudicone JM, Amatniek J, Marcus RN, Sheehan JJ (2014) A randomized controlled trial investigating the safety and efficacy of aripiprazole in the long-term maintenance treatment of pediatric patients with irri-tability associated with autistic disorder. J Clin Psychiatry 75(1):22–30

Fink M (2013) Rediscovering catatonia: the biography of a treatable syndrome. Acta Psych Scand 127(suppl 441):1–47

Fink M, Taylor M (2003) Catatonia: a clinician's guide to diagnosis and treatment. Cambridge University Press, Cambridge

Fink M, Taylor MA, Ghaziuddin N (2006) Catatonia in autistic spectrum disorders: a medical treatment algorithm. Int Rev Neurobiol 72:233–244

Frazier JA, Doyle R, Chiu S, Coyle JT (2002) Treating a child with Asperger's disorder and comor-bid bipolar disorder. Am J Psychiatry 159(1):13–21

Frühe B, Allgaier AK, Pietsch K, Baethmann M, Peters J, Kellnar S, Heep A, Burdach S, von Schweinitz D, Schulte-Körne G (2012) Children's depression screener (ChilD-S): develop-ment and validation of a depression screening instrument for children in pediatric care. Child Psychiatry Hum Dev 43:137–151

Ghaziuddin M, Greden J (1998) Depression in children with autism/pervasive developmental dis-order: a case-control family history study. J Autism Dev Disord 28(2):111–115

Ghaziuddin M, Alessi N, Greden JF (1995) Life events and depression in children with pervasive developmental disorders. J Autism Dev Disord 25(5):495–502

Ghaziuddin M, Ghaziuddin N, Greden J (2002) Depression in persons with autism: implications for research and clinical care. J Autism Dev Disord 32(4):299–306

Gotham K, Unruh K, Lord C (2014) Depression and its measurement in verbal adolescents and adults with autism spectrum disorder. Autism 10.

Gracious BL, Youngstrom EA, Findling RL, Calabrese JR (2002) Discriminative validity of a parent version of the young mania rating scale. J Am Acad Child Adolesc Psychiatry 41:1350–1359

Green J, Gilchrist A, Burton D, Cox A (2000) Social and psychiatric functioning in adolescents with Asperger Syndrome compared with conduct disorder. J Autism Dev Disord 30(4):279–293

Hallett V, Ronald A, Rijsdijk F, Happé F (2010) Association of autistic-like and internalizing traits during childhood: a longitudinal twin study. Am J Psychiatry 167(7):809–817

Hallett V, Ronald A, Rijsdijk F, Happé F (2012) Disentangling the associations between autistic-like and internalizing traits: a community based twin study. J Abnorm Child Psychol 40(5):815–827

Hamilton M (1960) A rating scale for depression. J Neurol Neurosurg Psychiatry 23:56–62

Hammen C (2005) Stress and depression. Ann Rev Clin Psychol 1:293–319

Hedley D, Young R (2006) Social comparison processes and depressive symptoms in children and adolescents with Asperger syndrome. Autism 10:139–153

Hellings JA, Weckbaugh M, Nickel EJ, Cain SE, Zarcone JR, Reese RM, Hall S, Ermer DJ, Tsai LY, Schroeder SR, Cook EH (2005) A double-blind, placebo-controlled study of valproate for aggression in youth with pervasive developmental disorders. J Child Adolesc Psychopharmacol 15(4):682–692

Helverschou SB, Bakken TL, Martinsen H (2009) The psychopathology in autism checklist (PAC): a pilot study. Res Aut Spectrum Disord 3:179–195

Henry CA, Nowinski L, Koesterer K, Ferrone C, Spybrook J, Bauman M (2014) Low rates of depressed mood and depression diagnoses in a clinic review of children and adolescents with autistic disorder. J Child Adolesc Psychopharmacol 24(7):403–406

Hofmann SG, Sawyer AT, Witt AA, Oh D (2010) The effect of mindfulness-based therapy on anxiety and depression: a meta-analytic review. J Consult Clin Psychol 78:169–183

Hofvander B, Delorme R, Chaste P, Nydén A, Wentz E, Ståhlberg O, Herbrecht E, Stopin A, Anckarsäter H, Gillberg C, Råstam M, Leboyer M (2009) Psychiatric and psychosocial problems in adults with normal-intelligence autism spectrum disorders. BMC Psychiatry 10:9–35

Hollander E, Chaplin W, Soorya L, Wasserman S, Novotny S, Rusoff J, Feirsen N, Pepa L, Anagnostou E (2010) Divalproex sodium vs placebo for the treatment of irritability in children and adolescents with autism spectrum disorders. Neuropsychopharmacology 35(4):990–998

Humphrey N, Lewis S (2008) 'Make me normal': the views and experiences of pupils on the autistic spectrum in mainstream secondary schools. Autism 12(1):23–46

Hurwitz R, Blackmore R, Hazell P, Williams K, Woolfenden S (2012) Tricyclic antidepressants for autism spectrum disorders (ASD) in children and adolescents. Cochrane Database Syst Rev 3, CD008372

Janusonis S (2005) Statistical distribution of blood serotonin as a predictor of early autistic brain abnormalities. Theor Biol Med Model 19:2–27

Jepsen MJ, Gray KM, Taffe JR (2012) Agreement in multi-informant assessment of behaviour and emotional problems and social functioning in adolescents with Autistic and Asperger's Disorder. Res Aut Spectrum Disord 6:1091–1098

Jiang HY, Qiao F, Xu XF, Yang Y, Bai Y, Jiang LL (2013) Meta-analysis confirms a functional polymorphism (5-HTTLPR) in the serotonin transporter gene conferring risk of bipolar disorder in European populations. Neurosci Lett 549:191–196

Joshi G, Biederman J, Wozniak J, Doyle R, Hammerness P, Galdo M, Sullivan N, Williams C, Brethel K, Woodworth KY, Mick E (2012) Response to second generation antipsychotics in youth with comorbid bipolar disorder and autism spectrum disorder. CNS Neurosci Ther 18(1):28–33

Joshi G, Biederman J, Petty C, Goldin RL, Furtak SL, Wozniak J (2013) Examining the comorbidity of bipolar disorder and autism spectrum disorders: a large controlled analysis of phenotypic and familial correlates in a referred population of youth with bipolar I disorder with and without autism spectrum disorders. J Clin Psychiatry 74(6):578–586

Kabat-Zinn J (1990) Full catastrophe living: using the wisdom of your body and mind to face stress, pain, and illness. Delacourt, New York

Kamburov A, Wierling C, Lehrach H, Herwig R (2009) ConsensusPathDB-a database for integrating human functional interaction networks. Nucleic Acids Res 37(Database issue):D623–D628

Kaufman J, Birmaher B, Brent D, Rao U, Flynn C, Moreci P, Williamson D, Ryan N (1997) Schedule for affective disorders and schizophrenia for school-age children-present and lifetime version (K-SADS-PL): initial reliability and validity data. J Am Acad Child Adolesc Psychiatry 36(7):980–988

Kepser LJ, Homberg JR (2015) The neurodevelopmental effects of serotonin: A behavioural perspective. Behav Brain Res 277:3–13

Kerestes R, Davey CG, Stephanou K, Whittle S, Harrison BJ (2013) Functional brain imaging studies of youth depression: a systematic review. Neuroimage Clin 4:209–231

Kim J, Szatmari P, Bryson S, Streiner DL, Wilson FJ (2000) The prevalence of anxiety and mood problems among children with autism and Asperger syndrome. Autism 4:117–132

Kimberly A (2014) Stigler psychopharmacologic management of serious behavioral disturbance in ASD. Child Adolesc Psychiatr Clin N Am 23:73–82

King BH (2000) Pharmacological treatment of mood disturbances, aggression, and self-injury in persons with pervasive developmental disorders. J Autism Dev Disord 30(5):439–445

Kirino E (2014) Efficacy and tolerability of pharmacotherapy options for the treatment of irritability in autistic children. Clin Med Insights Paediatr 8:17–30

Kovacs M (1982) The children's depression inventory: a self-rated depression scale of school-aged youngsters. University of Pittsburgh School of Medicine, Pittsburgh

Kuroda M, Kawakubo Y, Kuwabara H, Yokoyama K, Kano Y, Kamio Y (2013) A cognitive-behavioral intervention for emotion regulation in adults with high-functioning autism spectrum disorders: study protocol for a randomized controlled trial. Trials 23(14):231

Lainhart JE (1999) Psychiatric problems in individuals with autism, their parents and siblings. Int Rev Psychiatry 11:278–298

Lainhart JE, Folstein S (1994) Affective disorders in people with autism: a review of published cases. J Autism Dev Disord 24:587–601

Leyfer OT, Folstein SE, Bacalman S, Davis NO, Dinh E, Morgan J, Tager-Flusberg H, Lainhart JE (2006) Comorbid psychiatric disorders in children with autism: interview development and rates of disorders. J Autism Dev Disord 36:849–861

Little L (2002) Middle-class mothers' perceptions of peer and sibling victimization among children with Asperger's syndrome and nonverbal learning disorders. Issues Compr Pediatr Nurs 25(1):43–57

Lugnegård T, Unenge Hallerbäck M, Gillberg C (2011) Psychiatric comorbidity in young adults with a clinical diagnosis of Asperger syndrome. Res Dev Disabil 32(5):1910–1917

Magnuson KM, Constantino JN (2011) Characterization of depression in children with autism spectrum disorders. J Dev Behav Pediatr 32(4):332–340

Marcus RN, Owen R, Kamen L, Manos G, McQuade RD, Carson WH, Aman MG (2009) A placebo-controlled, fixed-dose study of aripiprazole in children and adolescents with irritability associated with autistic disorder. J Am Acad Child Adolesc Psychiatry 48(11):1110–1119

Matson JL, Boisjoli JA (2003) Autism spectrum disorders in adults with intellectual disability and comorbid psychopathology: scale development and reliability of the ASD-CA. Res Aut Spectrum Disord 2:276–287

Matson JL, Wilkins J (2008) Reliability of the autism spectrum disorders-comorbidity for children (ASD-CC). J Dev Phys Disabil 20:155–165

Matson JL, LoVullo SV, Rivet TT, Boisjoli JA (2009) Validity of the autism spectrum disorder-comorbid for children (ASD-CC). Res Aut Spectrum Disord 3:345–357

Mattila ML, Hurtig T, Haapsamo H, Jussila K, Kuusikko-Gauffin S, Kielinen M, Linna SL, Ebeling H, Bloigu R, Joskitt L, Pauls DL, Moilanen I (2010) Comorbid psychiatric disorders associated with Asperger syndrome/high-functioning autism: a community and clinic-based study. J Autism Dev Disord 40(9):1080–1093

Mazefsky CA, Kao J, Oswald DP (2011) Preliminary evidence suggesting caution in the use of psychiatric self-report measures with adolescents with high-functioning autism spectrum disorders. Res Aut Spectrum Disord 5(1):164–174

Mazurek MO (2014) Loneliness, friendship, and well-being in adults with autism spectrum disorders. Autism 18(3):223–232

Mazzone L, Curatolo P (2010) Conceptual and methodological challenges for neuroimaging studies of autistic spectrum disorders. Behav Brain Funct 9:6–17

Mazzone L, Ruta L, Reale L (2012) Psychiatric comorbidities in Asperger syndrome and high functioning autism: diagnostic challenges. Ann Gen Psychiatry 11(1):16

Mazzone L, Postorino V, De Peppo L, Fatta L, Lucarelli V, Reale L, Giovagnoli G, Vicari S (2013) Mood symptoms in children and adolescents with autism spectrum disorders. Res Dev Disabil 34(11):3699–3708

Mazzone L, Postorino V, Valeri G, Vicari S (2014) Catatonia in patients with autism: prevalence and management. CNS Drugs 28(3):205–215

McDougle CJ, Holmes JP, Bronson MR, Anderson GM, Volkmar FR, Price LH, Cohen DJ (1997) Risperidone treatment of children and adolescents with pervasive developmental disorders: a prospective open label study. J Am Acad Child Adolesc Psychiatry 36(5):685–693

Meyer RR (2013) A review of the serotonin transporter and prenatal cortisol in the development of autism spectrum disorders. Mol Autism 4(1):37

Mottolese R, Redouté J, Costes N, Le Bars D, Sirigu A (2014) Switching brain serotonin with oxytocin. Proc Natl Acad Sci U S A 111(23):8637–8642

Munesue T, Ono Y, Mutoh K, Shimoda K, Nakatani H, Kikuchi M (2008) High prevalence of bipolar disorder comorbidity in adolescents and young adults with high-functioning autism spectrum disorder: a preliminary study of 44 outpatients. J Affect Disord 111(2–3): 170–175

Myers K, Winters NC (2002) Ten-year review of rating scales. II: scales for internalizing disorders. J Am Acad Child Adolesc Psychiatry 41:634–659

Nonacs R, Cohen LS (2003) Assessment and treatment of depression during pregnancy: an update. Psychiatr Clin North Am 26(3):547–562

O'Brien G, Pearson J, Berney T, Barnard L (2001) Measuring behaviour in developmental disability: a review of existing schedules. Dev Med Child Neurol Suppl 87:1–72

Orinstein AJ, Helt M, Troyb E, Tyson KE, Barton ML, Eigsti IM, Naigles L, Fein DA (2014) Intervention for optimal outcome in children and adolescents with a history of autism. J Dev Behav Pediatr 35(4):247–256

Ozonoff S, Dawson G, McPartland J (2002) A parent's guide to Asperger syndrome and high-functioning autism. Guilford Press, New York

Pine DS, Guyer AE, Goldwin M, Towbin KA, Leibenluft E (2008) Autism spectrum disorder scale scores in pediatric mood and anxiety disorders. J Am Acad Child Adolesc Psychiatry 47(6):652–661

Politte LC, Henry CA, McDougle CJ (2014) Psychopharmacological interventions in autism spectrum disorder. Harv Rev Psychiatry 22(2):76–92

Pouw L, Rieffe C, Stockmann L, Gadow KD (2013) The link between emotion regulation, social functioning, and depression in boys with ASD. Res Aut Spectrum Disord 7:549–556

Poznanski EO, Mokros HB (1996) Children's depression rating scale, revised (CDRS-R) manual. Western Psychological Services Publishers and Distributors, Los Angeles

Radloff LS (1977) The CES-D scale: a self-report depression scale for research in the general population. Appl Psychol Meas 1:385–401

Ragunath P, Chitra R, Mohammad S, Abhinand P (2011) A systems biological study on the comorbidity of autism spectrum disorders and bipolar disorder. Bioinformation 7(3):102–106

Ramoz N, Cai G, Reichert JG, Corwin TE, Kryzak L, Smith CJ, Silverman JM, Hollander E, Buxbaum JD (2006) Family-based association study of TPH1 andTPH2 polymorphisms in autism. Am J Med Genet B Neuropsychiatr Genet 141 B(8):861–7

Reichow B, Steiner AM, Volkmar F (2012) Social skills groups for people aged 6 to 21 with autism spectrum disorders (ASD). Evid-Based Child Health 7:266–315

Rosenberg RE, Kaufmann WE, Law JK, Law PA (2011) Parent report of community psychiatric comorbid diagnoses in autism spectrum disorders. Autism Res Treat. 405849

Scherff A, Taylor M, Eley TC, Happé F, Charman T, Ronald A (2014) What causes internalising traits and autistic traits to co-occur in adolescence? A Community-Based Twin Study. J Abnorm Child Psychol 42:601–610

Shaffer D, Fisher P, Lucas CP, Dulcan MK, Schwab-Stone ME (2000) NIMH diagnostic interview schedule for children version IV (NIMH DISC-IV): description, differences from previous versions, and reliability of some common diagnoses. J Am Acad Child Adolesc Psychiatry 39(1):28–38

Siegel M, Beresford CA, Bunker M, Verdi M, Vishnevetsky D, Karlsson C, Teer O, Stedman A, Smith KA (2014) Preliminary investigation of lithium for mood disorder symptoms in children and adolescents with autism spectrum disorder. J Child Adol Psychopharmacol 24(7):399–402

Simonoff E, Pickles A, Charman T, Chandler S, Loucas T, Baird G (2008) Psychiatric disorders in children with autism spectrum disorders: prevalence, comorbidity, and associated factors in a population-derived sample. J Am Acad Child Adolesc Psychiatry 47(8):921–929

Simonoff E, Jones CR, Pickles A, Happé F, Baird G, Charman T (2012) Severe mood problems in adolescents with autism spectrum disorder. J Child Psychol Psychiatry 53(11): 1157–1166

Skeppar P, Thoor R, Sture A, Isakson A, Skeppar I, Persson B, Fitzgerald M (2013) Neurodevelopmental disorders with comorbid affective disorders sometimes produce psychiatric conditions traditionally diagnosed as schizophrenia. Clin Neuropsychiatr 10(3–4): 123–133

Sofronoff K, Attwood T, Hinton S, Levin I (2007) A randomized controlled trial of a cognitive behavioural intervention for anger management in children diagnosed with Asperger syndrome. J Autism Dev Disord 37:1203–1214

Spek AA, van Hama NC, Nyklıcek I (2013) Mindfulness-based therapy in adults with an autism spectrum disorder: a randomized controlled trial. Res Dev Dis 34:246–253

Spitzer RL, Williams JBW, Kroenke K, Linzer M, deGruy FVIII, Hahn SR et al (1994) Utility of a new procedure for diagnosing mental disorders in primary care: the PRIME-MD 1000 study. JAMA 272:1749–1756

Stachnik JM, Nunn-Thompson C (2007) Use of atypical antipsychotics in the treatment of autistic disorder. Ann Pharmacother 41(4):626–634

Stahlberg O, Soderstrom H, Rastam M, Gillberg C (2004) Bipolar disorder, schizophrenia, and other psychotic disorders in adults with childhood onset AD/HD and/or autism spectrum disorders. J Neural Transm 111(7):891–902

Sterling L, Dawson G, Estes A, Greenson J (2008) Characteristics associated with presence of depressive symptoms in adults with autism spectrum disorder. J Autism Dev Disord 38(6):1011–1018

Stewart ME, Barnard L, Pearson J, Hasan R, O'Brien G (2006) Presentation of depression in autism and Asperger syndrome: a review. Autism 10:103–116

Strang JF, Kenworthy L, Daniolos P, Case L, Wills MC, Martin A, Wallace GL (2012) Depression and anxiety symptoms in children and adolescents with autism spectrum disorders without intellectual disability. Res Autism Spectr Disord 6(1):406–412

Strauss C, Cavanagh K, Oliver A, Pettman D (2014) Mindfulness-based interventions for people diagnosed with a current episode of an anxiety or depressive disorder: a meta-analysis of randomized controlled trials. PLoS One 9(4), e96110

Takaoka K, Takata T (2007) Catatonia in high-functioning autism spectrum disorders: case report and review of literature. Psychol Rep 101:961–969

Tantam D (2000) Psychological disorder in adolescents and adults with Asperger syndrome. Autism 4:47–62

Teasdale JD, Segal ZV, Williams MG (1995) How does cognitive therapy prevent depressive relapse and why should attentional control (mindfulness training) help? Behav Res Ther 33:25–39

Thorson RT, Matson J (2012) Cutoff scores for the autism spectrum disorder – comorbid for children (ASD-CC). Res Aut Spectrum Disord 6:556–559

Towbin KE, Pradella A, Gorrindo T, Pine DS, Leibenluft E (2005) Autism spectrum traits in children with mood and anxiety disorders. J Child Adol Psychopharmacol 15(3):452–464

Troyb E, Orinstein A, Tyson K, Helt M, Eigsti IE, Stevens M, Fein D (2014) Academic abilities in children and adolescents with a history of autism spectrum disorders who have achieved optimal outcomes. Autism 18:233–243

Vannucchi G, Masi G, Toni C, Dell'Osso L, Erfurth A, Perugi G (2014) Bipolar disorder in adults with Asperger's syndrome: a systematic review. J Affect Disord 168:151–160

Veenstra-vanderweele J, Kim S, Lord C, Courchesne R, Akshoomoff N, Leventhal BL, Courchesne E, Cook EH Jr (2001) Transmission disequilibrium studies of the serotonin 5-HT 2A receptor gene (HTR2A) in autism. Am J Med Genet 114(3):277–283

Vickerstaff S, Heriot S, Wong M, Lopes A, Dossetor D (2007) Intellectual ability, self-perceived social competence and depressive symptomatology in children with high-functioning autistic spectrum disorders. J Autism Dev Disord 37(9):1647–1664

Voelbel GT, Bates ME, Buckman JF, Pandina G, Hendren RL (2006) Caudate nucleus volume and cognitive performance: are they related in childhood psychopathology? Biol Psychiatry 60(9):942–950

Weiss JA, Lunsky Y (2010) Group cognitive behaviour therapy for adults with Asperger syndrome and anxiety or mood disorder: a case series. Clin Psychol Psychother 17(5):438–446

Weissman A, Bates ME (2010) Increased clinical and neurocognitive impairment in children with autism spectrum disorders and comorbid bipolar disorder. Res Aut Spectrum Disord 4:670–680

Welner Z, Reich W, Herjanic B, Jung KG, Amado H (1987) Reliability, validity, and parent-child agreement studies of the diagnostic interview for children and adolescents (DICA). J Am Acad Child Adolesc Psychiatry 26(5):649–653

Whitehouse AJ, Durkin K, Jacquet E, Ziatas K (2009) Friendship, loneliness and depression in adolescents with Asperger's syndrome. J Adolesc 32(2):309–322

Wiggins JL, Peltier SJ, Bedoyan JK, Carrasco M, Welsh RC, Martinet DM, Lord C, Monk CS (2012) The impact of serotonin transporter genotype on default network connectivity in children and adolescents with autism spectrum disorders. Neuroimage Clin 2:17–24

Williamson S, Craig J, Slinger R (2008) Exploring the relationship between measures of self-esteem and psychological adjustment among adolescents with Asperger syndrome. Autism 12(4):391–402

Wing L (1996) The autistic spectrum: a guide for parents and professionals. Constable, London

Wing L, Shah A (2000) Catatonia in autistic spectrum disorders. Br J Psychiatry 176:357–362

Wozniak J, Biederman J, Faraone S, Frazier J, Kim J, Millstein R, Gershon J, Thornell A, Cha K, Snyder JB (1997) Mania in children with pervasive developmental disorder, revisited. J Am Acad Child Adolesc Psychiatry 36(11):1552–1559

Young RC, Biggs JT, Ziegler VE, Meyer DA (1978) A rating scale for mania: reliability, validity and sensitivity. Br J Psychiatry 133:429–435

Zhang H, Chen Z, Jia Z, Gong Q (2014) Dysfunction of neural circuitry in depressive patients with suicidal behaviors: a review of structural and functional neuroimaging studies. Prog Neuropsychopharmacol Biol Psychiatry 53:61–66

Zigmond AS, Snaith RP (1983) The hospital anxiety and depression scale. Acta Psychiatr Scand 67:361–370

Mirko Uljarevic, Heather Nuske, and Giacomo Vivanti

1   Introduction

Anxiety has been linked to autism spectrum disorder (ASD) since Leo Kanner and Hans Asperger first described this condition seven decades ago. Kanner (1943) provides a detailed report on a child whose behavior was "governed by an anxiously obsessive desire for the maintenance of sameness." For example, he would get very anxious if furniture was moved around, but then his anxiety would suddenly disappear when things were rearranged as they were previously. Other children described by Kanner would experience anxiety in response to loud sounds or mechanical noises. Asperger (1944) mentions anxiety in a different context, reporting that some of his patients would feel anxious as a consequence of being mercilessly bullied at school.

Clarifying the nature of the link between autism and anxiety is currently considered to be a priority in the field, as anxiety issues can interfere drastically with the ability to participate in home, school, and community activities, and might impact on the child and family well-being and quality of life above and beyond the core symptoms of ASD (Davis III et al. 2014; Pellecchia et al. 2015).

M. Uljarevic
La Trobe University, Melbourne, Australia
e-mail: G.Vivanti@latrobe.edu.au

H. Nuske
University of Pennsylvania, Philadelphia, USA

G. Vivanti (✉)
AJ Drexel Autism Institute, Drexel University, Philadelphia, USA
e-mail: giacomo.vivanti@drexel.edu

© Springer International Publishing Switzerland 2016   21
L. Mazzone, B. Vitiello (eds.), *Psychiatric Symptoms and Comorbidities in Autism Spectrum Disorder*, DOI 10.1007/978-3-319-29695-1_2

2   Prevalence

The existing research shows that individuals with ASD exhibit higher levels of anxiety compared to both typically developing individuals (Kim et al. 2000; Bellini 2004; Gadow et al. 2005; Lopata et al. 2010) and individuals from other clinical groups, including Down syndrome (Evans et al. 2005), conduct disorder (Green et al. 2000), specific language impairment (Gillott et al. 2001), Williams syndrome (Rodgers et al. 2012a), and learning disabilities (Gadow et al. 2005; Gillot and Standen 2007). Additionally, there is evidence that individuals with ASD experience anxiety levels that are comparable to those of clinically anxious non-ASD individuals (Russell and Sofronoff 2005; Farrugia and Hudson 2006).

Reported prevalence of anxiety in ASD has varied widely, with estimates ranging from 13.6 to 84.1 % (Bellini 2004; Bradley et al. 2004; Kim et al. 2000; Muris et al. 1998; Lidstone et al. 2014). A recent systematic review (van Steensel et al. 2011) has identified that clinically significant levels of anxiety were present in 39.6 % of a pooled sample of 2,121 individuals with ASD obtained from 31 studies. Although findings are inconsistent, the most frequent anxiety disorders in ASD appear to be specific phobias, generalized anxiety disorder, separation anxiety disorder, obsessive-compulsive disorder, and social phobia (Muris et al. 1998; Evans et al. 2005; Gadow et al. 2005; Weisbrot et al. 2005; de Bruin et al. 2007; Gillot and Standen 2007; Sukhodolsky et al. 2008).

In conclusion, anxiety appears to be more common in ASD than in both the general population and various clinical groups, with possibly up to 40 % of individuals in the autism spectrum presenting elevated levels of at least on anxiety subtype.

3   Phenomenology and Clinical Issues

In many autobiographical accounts of individuals with ASD, the experience of feeling anxious is described with reference to symptoms and feelings that resemble those occurring in the typical population. For example, Temple Grandin (1992) reports, "The feeling [of anxiety] was like a constant feeling of stage fright all the time. I had a pounding heart, sweaty palms, and restless movements. (…) For weeks I had horrible bouts of colitis. (…) I started waking up in the middle of the night with my heart pounding." Nevertheless, the manifestation of anxiety in ASD might present differently from its expression in individuals without an ASD or might be less apparent. Several factors might underlie these differences.

First, manifestations of the core features of ASD and anxiety symptoms overlap frequently, and this can make anxiety symptoms "invisible" (Kerns and Kendall 2014; Renno and Wood 2013). For example, social avoidance/withdrawal can be an expression of anxiety as well as a manifestation of the social communication impairment that characterizes ASD. Similarly, ritualistic behaviors are a known manifestation of anxiety but also an expression of the restricted and repetitive features that are pathognomonic of ASD. Therefore, an anxiety disorder that manifest with social avoidance and ritualistic behaviors, while easily identifiable in a child without ASD, can easily pass unnoticed in a child with ASD.

Additionally, even when manifestations of anxiety do not overlap with ASD symptoms, they can be less noticeable in the context of the clinical variability observed in ASD. As the range of behavioral manifestations associated with ASD is extremely large and heterogeneous, any atypical behavior in this population can be mistakenly interpreted as being a consequence of having ASD (for an example of diagnostic overshadowing, see Kanne 2013). For example, the presence of restlessness and phobias (two symptoms of anxiety that do not overlap with the characteristic features of ASD) in a child who has severe ASD might be seen as a behavioral manifestation of ASD, rather than anxiety (Helverschou and Martinsen 2011; Kerns et al. 2015).

Furthermore, individuals with ASD might present with idiosyncratic anxiety symptoms. For example, recent research (Mayes et al. 2013; Kerns and Kendall 2014) documented a high proportion of atypical anxiety symptoms, including unusual specific phobias (e.g., vacuum cleaners, toilets) and fears of change/novelty. However, it is unclear whether such symptoms are manifestations of anxiety or reflect aspects of the core symptoms of ASD.

Communication difficulties further complicate the picture, as many individuals with ASD do not have the communication skills necessary to express their experience of distress or discomfort verbally. This both affects the overt manifestations of anxiety and limits the possibility to ascertain the presence of anxiety symptoms, in particular in minimally verbal children.

In summary, despite the high prevalence of anxiety in the ASD population, there is still uncertainty in the field on how to best define the clinical presentation of anxiety in individuals with ASD. This reflects the clinical issues discussed above (overlap between core symptoms of the two conditions, diagnostic overshadowing, atypical symptoms that encompass elements of both conditions, and impact of core ASD impairments in symptom expression), as well as current lack of knowledge on the causal relationship between ASD and anxiety. The increased risk for anxiety in individuals with ASD might reflect a number of different scenarios (Mazefsky and Herrington 2014; Weisbrot et al. 2005; Wood and Gadow 2010). First, it is possible that individuals with ASD are anxious as the inevitable consequence of having to cope with social demands that are beyond their level of understanding. The difficulties in core social cognition processes such as mindreading (Baron-Cohen 1997) and action understanding (Vivanti et al. 2011), as well as in social-affiliative behaviors such as establishing and maintaining social relationships, might result in perceiving the social world as unpredictable, confusing, and ultimately anxiety-provoking. Other factors that might lead to increased risk for anxiety in ASD include restrictions to self-determination that are often experienced especially in lower functioning individuals (Carter et al. 2013) and peer rejection encountered by higher functioning individuals who are motivated by the desire of friendships and relationships. Moreover, hypersensitivity to sensory stimuli (e.g., loud noises) might lead to the development of aversion and subsequent phobic responses to situations (e.g., dogs barking, balloons popping, vacuum cleaners) that would not normally trigger such reactions in typical peers. While there is evidence supporting this scenario (Wood and Gadow 2010; Hollocks et al. 2014) if anxiety is the inevitable consequence of having ASD, then is not clear why not all individuals with ASD have anxiety.

An alternative explanation is that features that are not specific or pathognomonic of ASD, but co-occur frequently in this population, confer the increased risk of anxiety in ASD. For example, intellectual disability, depression, tic disorders, and obsessive-compulsive disorder are frequently associated both with ASD and anxiety. Issues in emotional regulation, which are very frequent in ASD, might also play a relevant role (Mazefsky et al. 2013). Thus the occurrence of anxiety in this population is likely to reflect the interplay between different, co-occurring risk factors.

Finally, it is possible that ASD and anxiety share a common etiology (see section on Neurobiological Bases (Sect. 6)).

4   Correlates of Anxiety in ASD

In the typical population, the presentation of anxious symptoms is tied to normative developmental periods and the challenges they bring (Warren and Sroufe 2004). It is therefore expected that separation anxiety and phobias of animals should be predominant in children aged 6–9 years, generalized anxiety symptoms and phobias regarding danger and death in children aged 10–13 years, and social anxiety in adolescents around ages 14–17 years. Several studies have supported this model. For example, Kashani and Orvaschel (1990) looked at the fear of social situations across three age groups. In a group of 8-year-old children, fear of social situations was reported in approximately 21.4 %; this rate increased to 45.75 % of 12 year olds and to 55.7 % of 17 year olds. Furthermore, "worrying about what others think about me" was reported by 38.6 % of 8 year olds and increased to 67.1 % in 12 and 17 year olds.

Following these findings, several studies have examined the role of age and developmental level in the expression of anxiety in autism, with some studies reporting that higher levels of anxiety are associated with cognitive ability (Weisbrot et al. 2005; Lecavalier et al. 2006; Mazurek and Kanne 2010) and increased age (Kuusikko et al. 2008; Davis III et al. 2010; Green et al. 2012). However, other studies have failed to find associations between anxiety, cognitive level (Mazefsky et al. 2011; Strang et al. 2012), and chronological age (e.g., Strang et al. 2012). It is important to emphasize that existing literature has predominantly focused on school-aged children and adolescents, with only few studies examining anxiety in very young children (Davis III et al. 2011a; Matson et al. 2010; Green et al. 2012) and adult populations (Bejerot et al. 2014; Gillott and Standen 2007). A recent study by Davis III et al. (2011a) compared the levels of anxiety in 131 toddlers (aged 17–36 months), children (aged 3–16 years), and adults (aged 20–65 years) diagnosed with ASD and found that anxiety increases from toddlerhood to childhood, decreases from childhood to young adulthood, but again increases from young adulthood into older adulthood. Although the study by Davis and colleagues provides an initial insight into how anxiety might change over the lifespan in individuals with ASD, it is necessarily limited by the use of different anxiety measures for different age groups and more importantly by its cross-sectional design.

Studies examining the relationship between overall autism severity and anxiety have yielded mixed results, with Mazurek and Keane (2010) finding a significant negative association between autism severity and anxiety levels and Lopata et al. (2010) reporting no significant association.

Although research on anxiety in non-ASD populations has consistently shown a link between impairments in language and communication and levels of anxiety (Beitchman et al. 2001; Bornstein et al. 2013), only a handful of studies have examined the relationship between the social communication impairments and anxiety in ASD, consistently reporting that anxiety symptoms are more common in children with stronger communication abilities (Davis III et al. 2011b, 2012; Sukhodolsky et al. 2008; Kerns et al. 2015). However, several authors (e.g., Strang et al. 2012; Sukhodolsky et al. 2008; Tsai 1996) have suggested that lower levels of anxiety in minimally verbal children with ASD might be a consequence of difficulties in communicating anxious symptoms rather than a true reflection of lower levels of anxiety in this subgroup.

In a recent study, Kerns et al. (2015) reported that individuals with ASD and co-occurring anxiety displayed more self-injury and depression than those with ASD alone. In the same study, co-occurring anxiety was associated with high levels of parental stress. Finally, studies in this field have consistently reported that elevated levels of anxiety are associated with both increased sensory modulation problems (Ben-Sasson et al. 2008; Green et al. 2012; Lidstone et al. 2014; Mazurek et al. 2013) and higher levels of repetitive behaviors (Sukhodolsky et al. 2008; Rodgers et al. 2012a, b; Gotham et al. 2013).

5   Diagnosis and Evaluation: Assessment Tools

The diagnosis of anxiety disorders in people with ASD is complicated by a number of factors. Firstly, as approximately 30 % of individuals with autism remain minimally verbal throughout their lifespan (Tager-Flusberg and Kasari 2013), ascertainment of anxiety symptoms in this subgroup must rely on information provided by parents, teachers, or other caregivers. Since secondhand accounts of anxious thoughts or behavior can be problematic due to common misconceptions or biases of the reporter, diagnosticians should exercise a healthy level of caution when interpreting this information. For example, repetitive patterns of play in a child with ASD may appear to their parent as a symptom of obsessive-compulsive disorder (OCD), though children with ASD usually enjoy engaging in these behaviors, whereas those with OCD do not (Turner-Brown et al. 2011).

Challenges exist also with respect to self-reports from verbally fluent people with autism, due to difficulties in interoception (the sense of one's own physiological state) as well as difficulties in verbal expression of emotional states, one aspect of alexithymia, which is present in 40–65 % of individuals with ASD (Berthoz and Hill 2005; Hill et al. 2004). Nevertheless, self-reports from the individual affected are an important source of information in assessing symptoms and tailoring treatment strategies on individual needs.

Use of behavioral monitoring and, where possible, direct observation is recommended to supplement self- or other reports of anxiety. Behavioral monitoring has the advantage of tracking the triggers of anxiety for a particular individual in natural settings and has been used in children without ASD (e.g., Hagopian et al. 1990). Where a specific trigger is known, direct observation may include a behavioral avoidance test (Dadds et al. 1994), a method which involves systematically assessing avoidant behavior associated with a particular phobia-inducing stimulus. Therefore, as with any diagnosis, diagnoses of anxiety in ASD are likely to be more accurate when information is integrated across multiple sources.

A second source of complexity in assessing anxiety in people with ASD is the already mentioned degree of overlap in behavioral symptoms between the two disorders, despite the distinction in their function and phenomenology.

Due to this apparent overlap in symptoms, there has been an effort over the last decade to design ASD-specific diagnostic and evaluation tools for anxiety disorders which examine the particular way in which these symptoms arise, manifest, and are maintained in ASD, including potentially unique contributions of sensory sensitivities, inherent difficulties in negotiating social interactions, and difficulties regulating emotions and behavior. For example, the Autism Comorbidity Interview (ACI; Leyfer et al. 2006) includes questions to establish the child's emotions and behavior at his/her best in order to establish a baseline. Another approach is to use diagnostic and evaluation protocols for anxiety disorders designed for other populations to diagnose anxiety in individuals with ASD. However, large-scale studies on the psychometric properties of such measures when applied to ASD populations are lacking and the overlap in symptoms may cause a clinician to make incorrect inferences on the person with ASD's scores on such measures. Tools that are currently used to assess anxiety symptoms in ASD are listed in Table 2.1. As only few of these instruments are designed specifically for use in ASD, and for some the reliability and validity is yet to be established in the full range of anxiety disorders, more research in this area is needed to establish best practices in evaluating the presence and severity of anxiety features occurring in ASD.

This reinforces the need for a multi-method analysis of anxiety in ASD, including parental, caregiver, and/or teacher report and direct observation. Future research should investigate the feasibility of adding physiological measures such as heart rate and skin conductance response as an additional source of information in diagnostic and assessment protocols.

6   Neurobiological Bases of Anxiety in ASD

The very few studies that have directly explored neural correlates of anxiety in ASD have exclusively focused on the potential role of amygdala dysregulation. Kleinhans et al. (2010) found that increased levels of social anxiety were associated with increased activation of right amygdala during an emotion recognition task.

Table 2.1 Anxiety Assessment Tools

Name (reference)	Reporter	Sub-scales	Designed for ASD?	Age group
Autism Comorbidity Interview-Present and Lifetime Version (ACI-PL; Leyfer et al. 2006)	Parent version	Panic disorders, separation anxiety, social phobia, specific phobia, generalized anxiety, and OCD	Yes and has been used in some studies (e.g., Leyfer et al. 2006; Mazefsky et al. 2011; Mazefsky et al. 2012)	5–17 years
Anxiety Disorder Interview Schedule for DSM-IV-Child and Parent Versions (ADIS; Silverman and Albano 1996)	Parent and child versions available	DSM-IV referenced scales	No, but studies on ASD have been conducted (e.g., Storch et al. 2012; Chalfant et al. 2007; Drahota et al. 2011; Sze and Wood 2007, 2008; White et al. 2009; Wood et al. 2009)	6–17 years
Diagnostic Interview Schedule for Children IV (DISC IV; Shaffer et al. 2000)	Parent version	Simple phobia, social phobia, agoraphobia, panic disorder, separation anxiety disorder, avoidant disorder of childhood or adolescence, overanxious disorder, and obsessive-compulsive disorder	No, but studies on ASD have been conducted (e.g., Leyfer et al. 2006; Muris et al. 1998)	Parent: 6–17 years Child: 11–17 years
Baby and Infant Screen for Children with Autistic Traits (BISCUIT; Matson, Boisjoli, and Wilkins 2007)	Parent version	Part 1 and part 3 evaluate the symptoms of ASD and externalizing symptoms, respectively. Part 2 assesses comorbid psychopathology including an anxiety/repetitive scale, among others	Yes and has been used in some studies (e.g., Davis et al. 2010, 2011a; Matson et al. 2010)	17–37 months
Autism Spectrum Disorders-Comorbid for Children (ASD-CC; Matson and Gonzalez 2007; Matson and Wilkins 2008)	Parent version	Worry/depressed, among other scales	Yes and has been used in some studies (e.g., Davis et al. 2011a, b; Hess et al. 2010; Worley and Matson 2010)	3–16 years

(continued)

Table 2.1 (continued)

Name (reference)	Reporter	Sub-scales	Designed for ASD?	Age group
Behavioral Assessment System for Children-2 (BASC-2; Reynolds and Kamphaus 2004)	Parent, teacher, and self-report	Anxiety, somatization, and internalizing, among other scales	No, but ASD norms included and studies on ASD have been conducted (e.g., Bellini 2004; Burnette et al. 2005; Meyer et al. 2006; Solomon et al. 2008; Lopata et al. 2010)	Preschool, 2–5 years; child, 6–11 years; and adolescent, 12–21 years
Spence Children's Anxiety Scale (SCAS)/Spence Preschool Anxiety Scale (Spence 1998)	Parent and child versions available	Generalized anxiety, social anxiety, obsessive-compulsive disorder, physical injury fears, and separation anxiety	No, but studies on ASD have been conducted (e.g., Murris et al. 1998; Gillott et al. 2001; Russell and Sofronoff 2005; Chalfant et al. 2007; Greenway and Howlin 2010)	7–19 years/3–6 years
Screening for Childhood Anxiety and Related Emotional Disorders (SCARED; Birmaher et al. 1997, 1999)	Parent and child versions available	Somatic/panic, generalized anxiety, separation anxiety, and social phobia	No, but a study on ASD has been conducted (e.g., Reaven et al. 2012)	8–18 years
Early Child Inventory-5 (ECI-5; Gadow and Sprafkin 1997)	Parent and teacher versions available	Generalized anxiety disorder, separation anxiety disorder, social phobia, posttraumatic stress disorder, simple phobia, OCD	No, but studies on ASD have been conducted (e.g., Weisbrot et al. 2005)	3–5 years
Multidimensional Anxiety Scale for Children (MASC; March et al. 1997)	Parent and child versions available	Somatic/panic, general anxiety, separation anxiety, social phobia, and school phobia	No, but studies on ASD have been conducted (e.g., Bellini 2004, 2006; Sze and Wood 2008; White et al. 2009; Wood et al. 2009)	4–19 years
Child Behavior Checklist (CBCL; Achenbach and Rescorla 2001):	Parent, teacher, and child versions available	Internalizing, anxious/depressed, somatic complaints, anxiety problems, somatic problems, among other scales	No, but studies on ASD have been conducted (e.g., Juranek et al. 2006; Kuusikko et al. 2008; Sze and Wood 2008)	1.5–5 years, 6–18 years

Diagnostic Assessment for the Severely Handicapped-II (DASH-II; Matson 1996)	Parent version	Overall anxiety scale, among other scales		33–80 years
Revised Children's Anxiety and Depression Scale (RCADS; Chorpita et al. 2005)	Self-report	Major depressive disorder, panic disorder, social phobia, separation anxiety disorder, generalized anxiety disorder, and obsessive-compulsive disorder	No, but studies on ASD have been conducted (e.g., Hallet et al. 2013; Sterling et al. 2015)	6–18 years
Psychopathology in Autism Checklist (PAC; Helvershou et al. 2009)	Staff/caregiver	Overall anxiety scale, among other scales	Yes	17–56 years

Juranek et al. (2006) reported that increased total and right (but not left) amygdala volume was associated with higher levels of anxiety (as measured by the Anxious/ Depressed subscale of the Child Behavior Checklist) in a sample of 49 individuals with ASD (mean chronological age, 7 years and 11 months; range, 3 years and 8 months to 14 years and 8 months).

As the neurobiology of ASD is still poorly understood, it is informative to turn to the large body of work that has explored the role of certain brain structures in the development and maintenance of anxiety in non-ASD populations. A large network of brain structures are involved in fear and anxiety (see Paulus and Stein 2006; Shin and Liberzon 2010 for excellent overviews). Among these, the amygdala, ventromedial prefrontal cortex, hippocampus, and insula play a critical role, both separately and through their complex set of mutual connections, in the processes of threat detection, emotional learning, interceptive awareness, and monitoring that have been suggested to be impaired in anxiety disorders.

Dysregulation of these brain structures might be linked to anxiety in ASD, as structural and functional abnormalities in the amygdala, hippocampus, ventromedial prefrontal cortex, and insula have been reported in ASD across a number of research studies and investigation techniques, including postmortem exploration (Bauman and Kempler 1985), structural neuroimaging (Aylward et al. 1999; Sparks et al. 2002), and functional neuroimaging (Dalton et al. 2005). Inconsistencies exist with respect to the nature of such abnormalities, with some studies finding enlarged amygdala volume (Howard et al. 2000; Sparks et al. 2002) and overactivity (Dalton et al. 2005) and other reduced volume (Aylward et al. 1999; Pierce et al. 2001) and hypo-activity (Green et al. 2000; Muris et al. 1998). Furthermore, studies have suggested structural and functional abnormalities of prefrontal cortical areas (see Kaiser et al. 2010) and insula (Menon and Udin 2010) in ASD. Despite this suggestive evidence, the role of these regions, individually and especially in terms of patterns of connectivity, has not been fully explored, and our understanding of the neurobiology of anxiety in ASD is currently indirect and limited.

7 Treatment of Anxiety in ASD

7.1 Non-medical Treatments

The most commonly used nonmedical treatments for anxiety disorders in ASD are those rooted in cognitive behavioral therapy (CBT). The Coping Cat series of interventions for children, adolescents, and adults with anxiety has been shown to be effective (Kendall 1994), with results maintained at 1 and 7 years post treatment (Kendall et al. 2008). An adapted version of this program has recently been applied to high-functioning youth with ASD with comparable efficacy (McNally Keehn et al. 2013), showing the promise of CBT-based strategies for treatment of anxiety in ASD. However, as the treatment procedures in this program place many demands on the child's cognitive skills and language comprehension, applicability of this program might be limited to the higher functioning end of the autism spectrum.

Emerging evidence suggests that behavioral strategies, such as the use of graduated exposure and positive reinforcement for approach behavior, could be effective for treating phobic avoidance in individuals in the spectrum, including those who are more severely affected (Jennett and Hagopian 2008). Importantly, a number of intervention programs for ASD, such as TEACCH (Treatment and Education of Autistic and Communication Handicapped Children; Mesibov et al. 2004) and SCERTS (Social Communication, Emotional Regulation, and Transactional Support; Prizant et al. 2006), include targeted procedures to address anxiety issues, such as the use of highly predictable routines to decrease stress and uncertainty and strategies to prevent and recover from emotion dysregulation.

Research on the effectiveness of comprehensive intervention and specific strategies to improve anxiety symptoms in individuals with ASD, especially those with associated learning impairments, is still at its infancy.

7.2 Pharmacological Treatments

Current guidelines suggest the use of the selective serotonin reuptake inhibitors (SSRIs) and the serotonin and noradrenaline reuptake inhibitors (SNRIs) as the agents of choice for the first-line pharmacotherapy on anxiety disorders due to relatively good efficacy and relatively low incidence of adverse effects (Baldwin et al. 2011).

Only a few studies have explored potential efficacy of pharmacological agents in treating anxiety in ASD. Namerow et al. (2003) and Couturier and Nicolson (2002) have reported some evidence for treatment efficacy of SSRIs on anxiety in ASD population, while the study by Martin et al. (2003) found no evidence of improvement in anxiety symptoms. Furthermore, all three studies have noted significant adverse effects. For example, in the Martin et al. study, 13 individuals (72 %) had at least 1 adverse effect during the course of the trial, and treatment for 3 participants had to be terminated due to the behavioral activation. Similarly Namerow et al. (2003) reported adverse effects such as headache, sedation, aggression, and agitation in five individuals.

Finally, Buitelaar et al. (1998) found that 16 of 22 individuals with ASD aged 6–17 years experienced a reduction of anxiety (on the Clinical Global Impressions Scale) after being treated with buspirone for a period of 6–8 weeks. Unlike with SSRIs, side effects of buspirone were relatively mild.

7.3 Novel Treatment Strategies

One novel approach to the treatment of anxiety in children involves the use of computer-based CBT interventions. Khanna and Kendall (2010) adapted the Coping Cat program into a computer program, Camp Cope-A-Lot, and found no differences in effectiveness between the computer program and individualized CBT in young children (without ASD). This implementation method has not yet been used in people with ASD who have clinical levels of anxiety.

Another somewhat promising avenue for novel treatments of anxiety in ASD is the use of biofeedback devices to increase emotional awareness and support development in interoception in this population. Bio-monitoring systems measure, amplify, and feedback information primarily from nervous system processes such as respiration, heart rate, muscle tension, skin temperature, blood flow, and blood pressure to the individual being monitored, thus promoting awareness of these processes to facilitate voluntary control over body and mind. Recent reviews on the use of biofeedback to treat anxiety have shown some positive effects, particularly when multiple channels of biofeedback are used (Wells et al. 2012). However, the findings on bio- or neuro-feedback in ASD have not shown any specific effects on anxiety, but rather on cognitive processes such as executive functioning (Kouijzer et al. 2009). Larger scale studies are needed to confirm these findings and establish effective protocols for individuals in the autism spectrum presenting with co-occurring anxiety symptoms.

8   Conclusions and Future Directions

While anxiety is very prevalent and causes significant impairments in the ASD population, research in this area is still in its infancy. A critical challenge for researchers and clinicians alike is the issue of whether anxiety is a manifestation of core autistic symptoms, a causally unrelated co-occurring condition, a consequence of the challenges faced by individuals with ASD in their social environment, or a combination of different factors. Dedicated research programs investigating typical and atypical anxiety symptom presentation, causal links between ASD and anxiety features, stability, and developmental changes in anxiety symptoms are needed to (1) reach a consensus around the concept of anxiety in ASD; (2) develop gold standard, multiaxial, developmentally sensitive assessment protocols for anxiety in ASD to complement standard evaluation procedures, and (3) identify treatment targets and develop individualized intervention programs to address this profoundly disabling comorbidity.

References

Achenbach TM, Rescorla LA (2001) Manual for the ASEBA School-Age Forms and Profiles. Burlington, VT: University of Vermont, Research Center for Children, Youth, and Families

Asperger H (1944) Die autistischen psychopathen in Kindersalten. Arch Psychiatr Nervenkrankenheiten 117:76–136

Aylward EH, Minshew NJ, Goldstein G, Honeycutt NA, Augustine AM, Yates KO, Barta PE, Pearlson GD (1999) MRI volumes of amygdala and hippocampus in non- mentally retarded autistic adolescents and adults. Neurology 53(9):2145–2150

Baldwin DS, Waldman S, Allgulander C (2011) Evidence-based pharmacological treatment of generalized anxiety disorder. Int J Neuropsychopharmacol 14(5):697–710

Baron-Cohen S (1997) Mindblindness: an essay on autism and theory of mind. MIT Press, Boston

Bauman M, Kemper TL (1985) Histoanatomic observations of the brain in early infantile autism. Neurology 35:866–874

Beitchman JH, Wilson B, Johnson CJ, Atkinson L, Young A, Adlaf E, Escobar M, Douglas L (2001) Fourteen-year follow-up of speech/language-impaired and control children: psychiatric outcome. J Am Acad Child Adolesc Psychiatry 40(1):75–82

Bejerot S, Eriksson JM, Mörtberg E (2014) Social anxiety in adult autism spectrum disorder. Psychiatry Res 220:705–707

Bellini S (2004) Social skill deficits and anxiety in high-functioning adolescents with autism spectrum disorders. Focus Autism Other Dev Disabil 19(2):78–86

Bellini S (2006) The development of social anxiety in adolescents with autism spectrum disorders. Focus on Autism and Other Developmental Disabilities, 21(3):138–145

Ben-Sasson A, Cermak SA, Orsmond GI, Tager-Flusberg H, Carter AS, Kadlec MB (2008) Sensory subgroups of toddlers with autism spectrum disorders: differences in internalizing symptoms. J Child Psychol Psychiatry 49(8):817–825

Berthoz S, Hill EL (2005) The validity of using self-reports to assess emotion regulation abilities in adults with autism spectrum disorder. Eur Psychiatry 20(3):291–298

Birmaher B, Brent DA, Chiappetta L, Bridge J, Monga S, Baugher M (1999) Psychometric properties of the Screen for Child Anxiety Related Emotional Disorders (SCARED): a replication study. J Am Acad Child Adolesc Psychiatry 38:1230–1236

Birmaher B, Khetarpal S, Brent D, Cully M, Balach L, Kaufman J, Neer MS (1997) The Screen for Child Anxiety Related Emotional Disorders (SCARED): scale construction and psychometric characteristics. J Am Acad Child Adolesc Psychiatry 36:545–553

Bornstein MH, Hahn CS, Suwalsky JT (2013) Language and internalizing and externalizing behavioral adjustment: developmental pathways from childhood to adolescence. Dev Psychopathol 25(3):857–878

Bradley EA, Summers JA, Wood HL, Bryson SE (2004) Comparing rates of psychiatric and behavior disorders in adolescents and young adults with severe intellectual disability with and without autism. J Autism Dev Disord 34:151–161

Buitelaar JK, van der Gaag RJ, van der Hoeven J (1998) Buspirone in the management of anxiety and irritability in children with pervasive developmental disorders: results of an open-label study. J Clin Psychiatry 59(2):56–59

Burnette CP, Mundy PC, Meyer JA, Sutton SK, Vaughan AE, Charak D (2005) Weak central coherence and its relations to theory of mind and anxiety in autism. J Autism Dev Disord 35:63–73

Carter EW, Lane KL, Cooney M, Weir K, Moss CK, Machalicek W (2013) Parent assessments of self-determination importance and performance for students with autism or intellectual disability. Am J Intellect Dev Disabil 118(1):16–31

Chalfant AM, Rapee R, Carroll L (2007) Treating anxiety disorders in children with high functioning autism spectrum disorders: a controlled trial. J Autism Dev Disord 37:1842–1857

Chorpita BF, Moffitt CE, Gray J (2005) Psychometric properties of the revised child anxiety and depression scale in a clinical sample. Behav Res Ther 43(3):309–322

Couturier JL, Nicholson R (2002) A retrospective assessment of citalopram in children and adolescents with pervasive developmental disorders. J Child Adolesc Psychopharmacol 12:243–248

Dadds MR, Rapee RM, Barrett PM (1994) Behavioral observation. In: Ollendick TH, King NJ, Yule W (eds) International handbook of phobic and anxiety disorders in children and adolescents. Plenum, New York, pp 349–364

Dalton KM, Nacewicz BM, Johnstone T, Schaefer HS, Gernsbacher MA, Goldsmith HH, Alexander AL, Davidson RJ (2005) Gaze fixation and the neural circuitry of face processing in autism. Nat Neurosci 8(4):519–526

Davis III TE, Fodstad JC, Jenkins WS, Hess JA, Moree BN, Dempsey T, … Matson JL (2010) Anxiety and avoidance in infants and toddlers with autism spectrum disorders: evidence for differing symptom severity and presentation. Res Autism Spectr Disord 4:305–313

Davis III TE, Hess JA, Moree BN, Fodstad JC, Dempsey T, Jenkins WS,… Matson J (2011a) Anxiety symptoms across the lifespan in people diagnosed with autistic disorder. Res Autism Spectr Disord 5:112–118

Davis III TE, Moree BN, Dempsey T, Reuther ET, Fodstad JC, Hess JA, … Matson JL (2011b) The relationship between autism spectrum disorders and anxiety: The moderating effect of communication. Res Autism Spectr Disord 5:324–329

Davis TE III (2012) Where to from here for ASD and anxiety? Lessons learned from child anxiety and the issue of DSM-5. Clin Psychol Sci Pract 19:358–363

Davis TE III, White SW, Ollendick TH (2014) Handbook of autism and anxiety. Springer, New York

de Bruin EI, Ferdinand RF, Meester S, De Nijs PFA, Verheij F (2007) High rates of psychiatric co-morbidity in PDD-NOS. J Autism Dev Disord 37:877–886

Drahota A, Wood JJ, Sze KM, Van Dyke M (2011) Effects of cognitive behavioral therapy on daily living skills in children with high-functioning autism and concurrent anxiety disorders. J Autism Dev Disord 41(3):257–265

Evans DW, Canavera K, Klinepeter FL, Taga K, Maccubbin E (2005) The fears, phobias and anxieties of children with autism spectrum disorders and Down syndrome: comparisons with developmentally and chronologically age matched children. Child Psychiatry Hum Dev 36:3–26

Farrugia S, Hudson J (2006) Anxiety in adolescents with Asperger syndrome: negative thoughts, behavioral problems, and life interference. Focus Autism Other Dev Disabil 21(1):25–35

Gadow KD, Sprafkin J (1997) Early Childhood Inventory-4 norms manual. Stony Brook, NY: Checkmate Plus

Gadow KD, DeVincent CJ, Pomeroy J, Azizian A (2005) Comparison of DSM-IV symptoms in elementary school-age children with PDD versus clinic and community samples. Autism 9:392–415

Gillot A, Furniss F, Walter A (2001) Anxiety in high-functioning children with autism. Autism 5:277–286

Gillott A, Standen PJ (2007) Levels of anxiety and sources of stress in adults with autism. J Intellect Disabil 11:359–370

Gotham K, Bishop SL, Hus V, Huerta M, Lund S, Buja A, Krieger A, Lord C (2013) Exploring the relationship between anxiety and insistence on sameness in autism spectrum disorders. Autism Res 6(1):33–41

Grandin, T (1992) An Inside View of Autism. In E. Schopler and G.B. Mesibov (eds), High-Functioning Individuals with Autism. New York: Plenum Press 105–26

Green SA, Ben-Sasson A, Soto TW, Carter AS (2012) Anxiety and sensory over-responsivity in toddlers with autism spectrum disorders: bidirectional effects across time. J Autism Dev Disord 42(6):1112–1119

Green J, Gilchrist A, Cox A (2000) Social and psychiatric functioning in adolescents with Asperger syndrome compared with conduct disorder. J Autism Dev Disord 30:279–293

Greenway R, Howlin P (2010) Dysfunctional attitudes and perfectionism and their relationship to anxious and depressive symptoms in boys with autism spectrum disorders. J Autism Dev Disord 40(10):1179–1187

Hagopian LP, Weist MD, Ollendick TH (1990) Cognitive-behavior therapy with an 11-year-old girl fearful of AIDS infection, other diseases, and poisoning: a case study. J Anxiety Disord 4:257–265

Hallett V, Ronald A, Colvert E, Ames C, Woodhouse E, Lietz S, Bolton P (2013) Exploring anxiety symptoms in a large-scale twin study of children with autism spectrum disorders, their co-twins and controls. Journal of Child Psychology and Psychiatry, 54(11), 1176–1185

Helverschou SB, Martinsen H (2011) Anxiety in people diagnosed with autism and intellectual disability: recognition and phenomenology. Res Autism Spectr Disord 5(1):377–387

Helvershou SB, Bakken TL, Martinsen H (2009) The psychopathology in autism (PAC): a pilot study. Res Autism Spectr Disord 3:179–195

Hess JA, Matson JL, Dixon DR (2010) Psychiatric symptom endorsements in children and adolescents diagnosed with autism spectrum disorders: a comparison to typically developing children and adolescents. J Dev Phys Disabil 22:485–496

Hill EL, Berthoz S, Frith U (2004) Brief report: cognitive processing of own emotions in individuals with autistic spectrum disorder and in their relatives. J Autism Dev Disord 34(2):229–235

Hollocks MJ, Jones CR, Pickles A, Baird G, Happé F, Charman T, Simonoff E (2014) The association between social cognition and executive functioning and symptoms of anxiety and depression in adolescents with autism spectrum disorders. Autism Res 7(2):216–228

Howard MA, Cowell PE, Boucher J, Broks P, Mayes A, Farrant A, ... Roberts N (2000) Convergent neuroanatomical and behavioral evidence of an amygdala hypothesis of autism. Neuroreport 11:2931–2935

Jennett HK, Hagopian LP (2008) Identifying empirically supported treatments for phobic avoidance in individuals with intellectual disabilities. Behav Ther 39:151–161

Juranek J, Filipek PA, Berenji GR, Modahl C, Osann K, Spence MA (2006) Association between amygdala volume and anxiety level: magnetic resonance imaging (MRI) study in autistic children. J Child Neurol 21(12):1051–1058

Kaiser MD, Hudac CM, Shultz S, Lee SM, Cheung C, Berken AM, Deen B, Pitskel NB, Sugrue DR, Voos AC, Saulnier CA, Ventola P, Wolf JM, Klin A, Vander Wyk BC, Pelphrey KA (2010) Neural signatures of autism. Proc Natl Acad Sci 107(49):21223–21228

Kanne S (2013) Diagnostic overshadowing. In: Encyclopedia of autism spectrum disorders. Springer, New York, pp 938–940

Kanner L (1943) Autistic disturbances of affective contact. Nerv Child 2:217–250

Kashani JH, Orvaschel H (1990) A community study of anxiety in children and adolescents. Am J Psychol 147:313–318

Kendall PC (1994) Treating anxiety disorders in children: results of a randomized clinical trial. J Consult Clin Psychol 62:100–110

Kendall PC, Hudson JL, Gosch E, Flannery-Schroeder E, Suveg C (2008) Cognitive-behavioral therapy for anxiety disordered youth: a randomized clinical trial evaluating child and family modalities. J Consult Clin Psychol 76:282–297

Kerns CM, Kendall PC (2014) Autism and anxiety: overlap, similarities, and differences. In: Handbook of autism and anxiety. Springer Cham Heidelberg New York Dordrecht London, pp 75–89

Kerns CM, Kendall PC, Zickgraf H, Franklin ME, Miller J, Herrington J (2015) Not to be overshadowed or overlooked: functional impairments associated with comorbid anxiety disorders in youth with ASD. Behav Ther 46(1):29–39

Khanna M, Kendall P (2010) Computer-assisted cognitive behavioral therapy for child anxiety: results of a randomized clinical trial. J Consult Clin Psychol 78(5):737–745

Kim JA, Szatmari P, Bryson SE, Streiner DL, Wilson FJ (2000) The prevalence of anxiety and mood problems among children with Autism and Asperger syndrome. Autism 4:117–132

Kleinhans NM, Richards T, Weaver K, Johnson LC, Greenson J, Dawson G, ... Alyward E (2010) Association between amygdala response to emotional faces and social anxiety in autism spectrum disorders. Neuropsychologia 48(12):3665–3670

Kouijzer MEJ, de Moor JMH, Gerrits BJL, Buitelaar JK, van Schie HT (2009) Long-term effects of neurofeedback treatment in autism. Res Autism Spectr Disord 3(2):496–501

Kuusikko S, Pollock-Wurman R, Jussila K, Carter AS, Mattila ML, Ebeling H, Pauls DL, Moilanen I (2008) Social anxiety in high-functioning children and adolescents with autism and Asperger syndrome. J Autism Dev Disord 38(9):1697–1709

Lecavalier L, Leone S, Wiltz J (2006) The impact of behaviour problems on caregiver stress in young people with autism spectrum disorders. J Intellect Disabil Res 50(3):172–183

Leyfer OT, Folstein SE, Bacalman S, Davis NO, Dinh E, Morgan J, Tager-Flusberg H, Lainhart JE (2006) Comorbid psychiatric disorders in children with autism: interview development and rates of disorders. J Autism Dev Disord 36:849–861

Lidstone J, Uljarević M, Sullivan J, Rodgers J, McConachie H, Freeston M, ... Leekam SR (2014) Relations among restricted and repetitive behaviors, anxiety and sensory features in children with autism spectrum disorders. Res Autism Spectr Disord 8(2):82–92

Lopata C, Toomey JA, Fox JD, Volker MA, Chow SY, Thomeer ML, Lee GK, Rodgers JD, McDonald CA, Smerbeck AM (2010) Anxiety and depression in children with HFASDs: symptom levels and source differences. J Abnorm Child Psychol 38(6):765–776

March JS (1997). Manual for multidimensional anxiety scale for children. Tonawanda, NY: Multi-Health System Inc

Martin A, Koenig K, Anderson G, Scahill L (2003) Low dose fluvoxamine treatment of children and adolescents with pervasive developmental disorders: A prospective, open-label study. J Autism Dev Disord 33(1):77–85

Matson JL, Benavidez DA, Compton LS, Paclawskyj T, Baglio C (1996) Characteristics of autism as assessed by the diagnostic assessment for the severely handicappated-II (DASH-II). Res Dev Disab 17, 135–143

Matson JL, Boisjoli JA, Wilkins J (2007) The Baby and Infant Screen for Children with aUtIsm Traits (BISCUIT). Disability Consultants, Baton Rouge

Matson JL, Gonzalez ML (2007) Autism spectrum disorders – comorbidity – child version. Disability Consultants, Baton Rouge

Matson JL, Hess JA, Boisjoli JA (2010) Comorbid psychopathology in infants and toddlers with autism and pervasive developmental disorders – not otherwise specified (PDD-NOS). Res Autism Spectr Disord 4(2):300–304

Matson JL, Wilkins J (2008) Reliability of the Autism Spectrum Disorders-Comorbid for Children (ASD-CC). J Dev Phys Disabil 20(4):327–336. doi:10.1007/s10882-008-9100-1

Mayes SD, Calhoun SL, Aggarwal R, Baker C, Mathapati S, Molitoris S, Mayes RD (2013) Unusual fears in children with autism. Res Autism Spectr Disord 7(1):151–158

Mazefsky CA, Herrington J (2014) Autism and anxiety: etiologic factors and transdiagnostic processes. In: Handbook of autism and anxiety. Springer International Publishing, pp 91–103

Mazefsky CA, Kao J, Oswald DP (2011) Preliminary evidence suggesting caution in the use of psychiatric self-report measures with adolescents with high-functioning autism spectrum disorders. Res Autism Spectr Disord 5:164–174

Mazefsky CA, Herrington J, Siegel M, Scarpa A, Maddox BB et al (2013) The role of emotion regulation in autism spectrum disorder. J Am Acad Child Adolesc Psychiatry 52:679–688

Mazefsky CA, Oswald DP, Day TN, Eack SM, Minshew NJ, Lainhart JE (2012) ASD, a psychiatric disorder, or both? Psychiatric diagnoses in adolescents with high-functioning ASD. J Clin Child Adolesc Psychol 41(4):516–523

Mazurek MO, Kanne SM (2010) Friendship and internalizing symptoms among children and adolescents with ASD. J Autism Dev Disabil 40(12):1512–1520

Mazurek MO, Vasa RA, Kalb LG, Kanne SM, Rosenberg D, Keefer A, Murray DS, Freedman B, Lowery LA (2013) Anxiety, sensory over-responsivity, and gastrointestinal problems in children with autism spectrum disorders. J Abnorm Child Psychol 41(1):165–176

McNally Keehn RH, Lincoln AJ, Brown MZ, Chavira DA (2013) The coping cat program for children with anxiety and autism spectrum disorder: a pilot randomized controlled trial. J Autism Dev Disord 43(1):57–67

Menon V, Udin LQ (2010) Saliency, switching, attention and control: a network model of insula function. Brain Struct Funct 214(5–6):655–667

Mesibov GB, Shea V, Schopler E (2004) The TEACCH approach to autism spectrum disorders. New York: Springer Science & Business Media

Meyer JA, Mundy PC, van Hecke AV, Durocher JS (2006) Social attribution processes and comorbid psychiatric symptoms in children with Asperger syndrome. Autism 10(4):383–402

Muris P, Steerneman P, Merckelbach H, Holdrinet I, Meesters C (1998) Comorbid anxiety symptoms in children with pervasive developmental disorders. J Anxiety Disord 12:387–393

Namerow LB, Prakash T, Bostic JQ, Prince J, Monuteaux AC (2003) Use of citalopram in pervasive developmental disorders. J Dev Behav Pediatr 24:104–108

Paulus MP, Stein MB (2006) An insular view of anxiety. Biol Psychiatry 60:383–387

Pellecchia M, Connell JE, Kerns CM, Xie M, Marcus SC, Mandell DS (2015) Child characteristics associated with outcome for children with autism in a school-based behavioral intervention. Autism 1362361315577518

Pierce K, Muller RA, Ambrose J, Allen G, Courchesne E (2001) Face processing occurs outside the fusiform 'face area' in autism: evidence from functional MRI. Brain 124:2059–2073

Prizant B, Wetherby A, Rubin E, Laurent A, Rydell P (2006) The SCERTS® model: a comprehensive educational approach for children with autism spectrum disorders, vol 1 and 2. Paul H. Brookes, Baltimore

Reaven J, Blakeley-Smith A, Leuthe E, Moody E, Hepburn S (2012) Facing your fears in adolescence: cognitive-behavioral therapy for high-functioning autism spectrum disorders and anxiety. Autism Res Treat. doi: 10.1155/2012/423905

Renno P, Wood JJ (2013) Discriminant and convergent validity of the anxiety construct in children with autism spectrum disorders. J Autism Dev Disord 43(9):2135–2146

Reynolds CR, Kamphaus RW (2004) Manual: behavior assessment system for children, 2nd edn. American Guidance Service, Circle Pines

Rodgers J, Riby DM, Janes E, Connolly B, McConachie H (2012a) Anxiety and repetitive behaviours in autism spectrum disorders and Williams syndrome: a cross-syndrome comparison. J Autism Dev Disord 42(2):175–180

Rodgers J, Glod M, Connolly B, McConachie H (2012b) The relationship between anxiety and repetitive behaviours in autism spectrum disorders. J Autism Dev Disord 42(11):2404–2409

Russell E, Sofronoff K (2005) Anxiety and social worries in children with Asperger syndrome. Aust N Z J Psychiatry 39:633–638

Shaffer D, Fisher P, Lucas CP, Dulcan MK, Schwab-Stone ME (2000) Diagnostic interview schedule for children version IV (DISC-IV): description, differences from previous versions, and reliability of some common diagnoses. J Am Acad Child Adolesc Psychiatry 39(1):28–38

Shin LM, Liberzon I (2010) The neurocircuitry of fear, stress, and anxiety disorders. Neuropsychopharmacology 35(1):169–191

Silverman W, Albano AM (1996) Manual for the anxiety disorders interview schedule for DSM-IV: child and parent versions. Psychological Corporation, San Antonio

Solomon M, Ozonoff S, Carter C, Caplan R (2008) Formal thought disorder and the autism spectrum: relationship between symptoms, executive control, and anxiety. J Autism Dev Disord 38:1474–1484

Sparks BF, Friedman SD, Shaw DW, Aylward EH, Echelard D, Artru AA, Maravilla KR, Giedd JN, Munson J, Dawson G, Dager SR (2002) Brain structural abnormalities in young children with autism spectrum disorder. Neurology 59:184–192

Spence SH (1998) A measure of anxiety symptoms among children. Behav Res Ther 36(5):545–566

Sterling L, Renno P, Storch EA, Ehrenreich-May J, Lewin AB, Arnold E, Lin E, Wood J (2015) Validity of the Revised Children's Anxiety and Depression Scale for youth with autism spectrum disorders. Autism. 2015 Jan;19(1):113–7. doi: 10.1177/1362361313510066

Storch EA, May JE, Wood JJ, Jones AM, De Nadai AS, Lewin AB, Arnold EB, Murpy TK (2012) Multiple informant agreement on the anxiety disorders interview schedule in youth with autism spectrum disorders. J Child Adolesc Psychopharmacol 22(4):292–299

Strang JF, Kentworthy L, Daniolos P, Case L, Willis MC, Martin A, Wallace GL (2012) Depression and anxiety symptoms in children and adolescents with autism spectrum disorders without intellectual disability. Res Autism Spectr Disord 6:406–412

Sukhodolsky DG, Scahill L, Gadow KD, Arnold LE, Aman MG, McDougle CJ, Tierney E, Williams White S, Lecavalier L, Vitiello B (2008) Parent-rated anxiety symptoms in children with pervasive developmental disorders: frequency and association with core autism symptoms and cognitive functioning. J Abnorm Child Psychol 36(1):117–128

Sze KM, Wood JJ (2007) Cognitive behavioral treatment of comorbid anxiety disorders and social difficulties in children with high functioning autism: a case report. J Contemp Psychother 37:133–143

Sze KM, Wood JJ (2008) Enhancing CBT for the treatment autism spectrum disorders and concurrent anxiety. Behav Cogn Psychother 36:403–409

Tager-Flusberg H, Kasari C (2013) Minimally verbal school-aged children with autism spectrum disorder: the neglected end of the spectrum. Autism Res 6(6):468–478

Tsai LY (1996) Brief report: comorbid psychiatric disorders of autistic disorder. J Autism Dev Disord 26:159–164

Turner-Brown LM, Lam KS, Holtzclaw TN, Dichter GS, Bodfish JW (2011) Phenomenology and measurement of circumscribed interests in autism spectrum disorders. Autism 15(4):437–456

van Steensel FJ, Bogels SM, Perrin S (2011) Anxiety disorders in children and adolescents with autistic spectrum disorders: a meta-analysis. Clin Child Fam Psychol Rev 14:302–317

Vivanti G, McCormick C, Young GS, Abucayan F, Hatt N, Nadig A, Ozonoff S, Rogers SJ (2011) Intact and impaired mechanisms of action understanding in autism. Dev Psychol 47(3):841

Warren SL, Sroufe LA (2004) Developmental issues. In: Ollendick TH, March JS (eds) Phobic and anxiety disorders in children and adolescents: a clinicians guide to effective psychosocial and pharmacological interventions. Oxford University Press, New York, pp 92–115

Weisbrot DM, Gadow KD, DeVincent CJ, Pomeroy J (2005) The presentation of anxiety in children with pervasive developmental disorders. J Child Adolesc Psychopharmacol 15:477–496

Wells R, Outhred T, Heathers JAJ, Quintana DS, Kemp AH (2012) Matter over mind: a randomised-controlled trial of single-session biofeedback training on performance anxiety and heart rate variability in musicians. PLoS One 7(10):e46597

White SW, Oswald D, Ollendick T, Scahill L (2009) Anxiety in children and adolescents with autism spectrum disorders. Clin Psychol Rev 29:216–229

Wood JJ, Gadow KD (2010) Exploring the nature and function of anxiety in youth with autism spectrum disorders. Clin Psychol Sci Pract 17(4):281–292

Wood JJ, Drahota A, Sze K, Har K, Chiu K, Langer DA (2009) Cognitive behavioral therapy for anxiety in children with autism spectrum disorders: a randomized, controlled trial. J Child Psychol Psychiatry 50(3):224–234

Worley JA, Matson JL, Sipes M, Koziowski AM (2010) Prevalence of autism spectrum disorders in toddlers receiving early intervention services. Res Autism Spectr Disord 5:920–925

Repetitive Behavior in Children with Autism Spectrum Disorder: Similarities and Differences with Obsessive-Compulsive Disorder

Lawrence Scahill and Saankari A. Challa

1   Introduction

Restrictive interests and repetitive behavior are defining features of autism spectrum disorder (ASD) (American Psychiatric Association 2013). The types of repetitive behaviors and restrictive interests vary widely in children with ASD from motor stereotypy to intense interests in unusual topics such as fans, air conditions, or television court shows (Bodfish et al. 2000; Lam and Aman 2007; Turner-Brown et al. 2011; Honey et al. 2012a; Bishop et al. 2013; Scahill et al. 2014). Although essential for the diagnosis of ASD, restricted interests and repetitive behavior (RRBs) may not be pressing problems in all cases. Heterogeneity of symptom types and severity of RRBs in ASD raise several challenges for diagnosis and treatment planning (Honey et al. 2012b; Scahill et al. 2015a). For example, bedtime rituals and favorite objects (special blankets or a favorite nightgown) are common in typically developing young children (Leekam et al. 2007; Arnott et al. 2009). In clinical practice, depending on the age of the child, it may be difficult to distinguish normal ritualistic behavior from abnormal RRBs. Repetitive behaviors are also central characteristics of obsessive-compulsive disorder (OCD) and Tourette syndrome. In addition, repetitive behaviors are often observed in children with developmental disabilities due to genetic syndromes, adults with schizophrenia, and adults with dementia (Moss et al. 2009; Morrens et al. 2006; Cipriani et al. 2013). These observations serve as a reminder that repetitive behavior in humans has an extraordinary range and is unlikely to have a single explanation (Lewis and Kim 2009; John et al. 2010).

Our understanding of repetitive and stereotypic behaviors in neurodevelopmental and psychiatric disorders has been informed by animal models on habit learning

L. Scahill (✉) • S.A. Challa
Department of Pediatrics, Marcus Autism Center, Emory University School of Medicine, Atlanta, GA, USA
e-mail: lawrence.scahill@emory.edu

© Springer International Publishing Switzerland 2016   39
L. Mazzone, B. Vitiello (eds.), *Psychiatric Symptoms and Comorbidities in Autism Spectrum Disorder*, DOI 10.1007/978-3-319-29695-1_3

(Berridge et al. 2005; de Wit and Dickinson 2009). A large body of preclinical data provides insight on the transition from goal-directed, reward-based behavior to automatic behavior (habit). When the reward-based behavior becomes habitual, it will persist even in the absence of reward (reward devaluation). Animal models suggest that the transition from goal-directed behavior to "automatic" behavior involves a shift in specific cortico-basal ganglia neural pathways (Alexander et al. 1986; Graybiel 2008). Given the wide range of RRBs in children with ASD and the potentially overlapping repetitive behaviors in children with OCD and Tourette syndrome, however, habit learning from preclinical models may not provide sufficient explanation for the phenomenon.

This chapter examines the similarities and differences of repetitive behavior in children with ASD and OCD. Examination of similarities and differences may help clinicians disentangle the repetitive behaviors attributable to OCD from those attributable to ASD, plan treatment and monitor progress. We begin with a brief deconstruction of comorbidity as it applies to ASD and OCD.

2 Comorbidity

Morbidity is a departure from a healthy state and is roughly equivalent to the disability caused by a symptom, syndrome, or disease. The term comorbidity implies the presence of two (or more) distinct conditions that are separately contributing to overall impairment. The boundaries between psychiatric conditions can be imprecise. This imprecision raises several questions about simple co-occurrence versus symptom overlap or the presence of a combined syndrome. For example, the co-occurrence of attention-deficit hyperactivity disorder (ADHD) and conduct disorder has long been proposed to represent an etiologically separate subgroup of ADHD (Banaschewski et al. 2003). If so, it would be inaccurate to consider conduct disorder as a comorbid condition with ADHD. Hyperactivity, impulsiveness, and distractibility are common in children with ASD (Gadow et al. 2006; Simonoff et al. 2008). In Diagnostic and statistical manual of mental disorders-text revised (DSM-IV-TR) however, clinicians were advised against giving a separate diagnosis of ADHD in line with the notion that the symptoms of ADHD could be explained by ASD (American Psychiatric Association 2000). Diagnostic and Statistical Manual of Mental Disorders, 5th edition, (DSM-5) has dropped this convention. Based on DSM-5, the presence of hyperactivity, impulsiveness, and distractibility in a child with ASD would be considered comorbid ADHD (American Psychiatric Association 2013). Here again, there is evidence that ADHD and ASD may have shared underlying genetic risk (Reiersen et al. 2007). There is also ongoing debate about whether anxiety disorders are separate from ASD or directly or indirectly caused by ASD or whether anxiety disorders are somehow blended with ASD (Kerns and Kendall 2012; Lecavalier et al. 2014). Discussion on co-occurrence versus overlap of OCD and ASD is not new and is not resolved (Baron-Cohen 1989; McDougle et al. 1995; Scahill et al. 2014). Among the phenomenological and conceptual problems inherent in this longstanding discussion is the simple fact that repetitive behaviors are central to the definition of both disorders.

3 Prevalence of OCD in ASD

The prevalence of OCD in the general population of children and adolescent is estimated to be between 2 % and 4 % with most studies leaning toward the lower end of this range (Geller 2006). Reports on the prevalence of OCD in children with ASD provide a stunning range of estimates from 2.6 % to 37.2 % (van Steensel et al. 2011). This wide range of estimates is due to differences in the source and size of the sample as well as the assessment methods used. For example, several studies included only higher functioning children. Sample sizes ranged from 20 to 300. Some studies used structured interviews; others used parent report on rating scales. Using a fixed-effect model in their meta-analysis, van Steensel and colleagues (2011) reported a 12.5 % prevalence of OCD in children with ASD. This estimate is clearly higher than the prevalence of OCD in the general population of children, but is substantially lower than the estimated co-occurrence of ADHD or other anxiety disorders in children with ASD (Simonoff et al. 2008).

4 Repetitive Behavior in OCD

Obsessive-compulsive disorder is defined by the presence of recurrent intrusive thoughts or worries, repetitive behaviors, or both. In order to meet the current diagnostic criteria for OCD in DSM-5, the obsessions and/or compulsions must be time consuming and cause marked distress or impairment. Intrusive thoughts or images (obsessions) are often accompanied by anxiety that may be temporarily relieved by performing intentional repetitive behaviors (compulsions). The sequence of obsessional worry (e.g., harm coming to the self or family) and rising anxiety, followed by anxiety reduction and by the compulsive behavior (e.g., checking), is the historical basis for classifying OCD as an anxiety disorder. In addition to anxiety caused by obsessions, compulsive behavior in children with OCD may be driven by a need to achieve a sense of completion rather than a clear-cut obsession (Geller 2006; Scahill et al. 2003). In DSM-5, OCD has been removed from anxiety disorders and placed with body dysmorphic disorder, trichotillomania, excoriation (skin-picking) disorder, and hoarding disorder under the rubric of obsessive-compulsive and related disorders. There is incomplete consensus on this new category in DSM-5 and findings from a large twin study do not fully support the position that these disorders are etiologically related (Monzani et al. 2014). In that study, Monzani and colleagues (2014) proposed that trichotillomania and skin-picking disorder appear to share genetic influences that are separate from OCD. Thus, the model of rising anxiety and temporary anxiety reduction should not be dismissed in favor of lumping disorders by virtue of repetitive behavior alone.

Common obsessions in children include recurring worries about contamination, harm coming to the self or family members, and abnormal need for symmetry. Common compulsions include handwashing, other cleaning rituals, touching in complex patterns, and repeating routine activities such as moving back and forth across a doorway (Rettew et al. 1992; Scahill et al. 2003; Geller 2006). Children with OCD usually describe their worries as nagging, unpredictable, unpleasant, and unwanted. Similarly, compulsions are unwelcomed behaviors that the child feels obliged to perform. Given the unwanted nature of obsessions and compulsions in OCD, affected children describe them as distressing and difficult to resist despite effort.

The connection between obsession and compulsion is often clear. The child who fears germ contamination may engage in compulsive handwashing. In other cases, the connection is remote. The child may describe the need to repeat a motor sequence such as bending down and touching the ground three times to prevent harm to a family member. Younger children may be unable to articulate that the behavior is unrelated to protect the family member. By contrast, adolescents may clearly state that the compulsive habit is unrelated and likely ineffective, yet they will perform the ritual "just in case." In still other cases of youth with OCD, repetitive behaviors are not connected to harm reduction. The child may describe touching in complex patterns or repeating a routine behavior (putting a key in and out of a lock several times before turning it) in order to avert a deep sense of physical discomfort. Even with the recognition that the behavior is unnecessary, the child may report that it is easier to perform the ritual than wrestle with the internal discomfort. Each of these examples reflects a negative reinforcement model in that the behavior is followed by decreased anxiety, doubt, or discomfort. For example, the child with compulsive handwashing may describe that the handwashing as necessary to reduce contamination, but it is the reduction in anxiety that reinforces the repetitive behavior. The child who touches the floor three times, six times, or nine times may do so to relieve feelings of doubt about an unrelated threat (for discussion of OCD phenomenology in children, see Rettew et al. 1992; Scahill et al. 2003; Geller 2006; Piacentini 2008).

To break down the apparent heterogeneity of OCD, several investigators have used factor analysis to build a basis for a dimensional approach that would classify OCD subtypes (Leckman et al. 1997; Rosario-Campos et al. 2006; Mataix-Coles et al. 2005; Miguel et al. 2005). Replicated symptom clusters include: (1) aggression and checking, (2) symmetry and ordering/arranging, (3) contamination and cleaning, and (4) hoarding. The replication of these factors across different samples supports the dimensional model of OCD rather than the broad categories of obsessions and compulsions. For example, contamination worries and washing rituals may provide a coherent clinical picture for establishing baseline severity and change with treatment – rather than considering obsessional worry as separate from the compulsive behavior. The dimensional schema may also be influenced by age (Diniz et al. 2004). In children, the onset of compulsions may precede the onset of obsessions or, perhaps, the child's ability to describe the obsession (Scahill et al. 2003). Children may engage in "tic-like" compulsion such as touching, tapping, blinking in patterns, and repeating routine activities such as opening and closing cupboard doors. These tic-like compulsions are more common in children with OCD with a history of tics and, in some cases, may be difficult to distinguish from complex tics (Leckman et al. 2001). The application of the dimensional approach to phenotypic characterization of subjects with OCD may be useful in neuroimaging studies, family history, and gene association studies and studies on moderators of treatment (Nestadt et al. 2002; Rauch and Jeike 1993; Monzani et al. 2014; Miguel et al. 2005; Rosario-Campos et al. 2006).

In summary, OCD in its paradigmatic form is characterized by the intrusion of unwanted thoughts that increase anxiety. The compulsive ritual reduces anxiety and, consequently, the behavior is reinforced. There is growing evidence that OCD is manifested by symptom clusters that may represent subtypes. The category of obsessive-compulsive and related disorders (including OCD, body dysmorphic disorder, hoarding, trichotillomania, excoriation) proposed in DSM-5 is not uniformly accepted and may not stand the test of time (American Psychiatric Association 2013).

5   Repetitive Behavior in ASD

As noted above, RRBs in children with ASD vary in type and severity. Repetitive behaviors range from stereotyped motor behaviors such as hand flapping, spinning, rocking, shaking fingers in front of the eyes, and repetitive self-injury. Repetitive behaviors may also involve more complex behaviors such as repeating phrases from movies, watching the same video segment over and over, lining up toys, and insistence on following routines in everyday living (e.g., eating, getting dressed or ready for bed in ritualized sequence) (Bodfish et al. 2000; Lam et al. 2008; Mirenda et al. 2010; Bishop et al. 2013; Scahill et al. 2014). Restricted interests may include fans, leaf blowers, car models, train schedules, or historical facts and figures (Turner-Brown et al. 2011). These restricted interests may meet the dictionary definition of obsession – but are not the same as unwanted and bothersome thoughts in OCD. In addition to time spent with such preoccupations, children with ASD may engage repeated questioning of others about the topic or expounding on it far beyond the listener's interest. This range of RRBs has been classified as higher and lower order behaviors. Lower order behaviors include motor stereotypy and other seemingly involuntary behaviors (Turner 1999). By contrast, higher order behaviors include what appear to be more deliberate activities. This broad categorization has been examined and reevaluated resulting in three to five categories. A factor analysis of the Autism Diagnostic Interview-Revised identified three subtypes: repetitive motor behaviors, insistence on sameness, and circumscribed interests (Lam et al. 2008). Based on expert opinion, the World Health Organization (WHO 2007) designated four subtypes: (a) preoccupations with part objects or nonfunctional elements of materials, (b) stereotyped and repetitive motor mannerisms, (c) preoccupations or circumscribed patterns of interest, and (d) adherence to specific nonfunctional routines or rituals (WHO 2007; Honey et al. 2012a, b). Factor analysis of the 43-item Repetitive Behavior Scale-Revised has yielded five factors: stereotyped behavior, self-injurious behavior (skin picking, biting self), compulsive behavior (ordering and arranging objects, counting, touching, and tapping), ritualistic/sameness behavior (insisting on certain order to eating or sleeping, insisting on arrangement of furniture or objects), and restricted interests (Lam and Aman 2007; Mirenda et al. 2010; Bishop et al. 2013).

In contrast to obsessive-compulsive symptoms in children with OCD, repetitive behaviors may not cause distress for children with ASD. Although the purpose of RRBs in children with ASD is not always clear, many children appear to have a strong drive to perform these behaviors (Honey et al. 2012a; Scahill et al. 2014). In some children, repetitive behavior such as hand flapping may increase during periods of anxiety or excitement (Bearss et al. 2015). In other cases, repetitive rocking may be used to reduce high levels of arousal or serve as a form of self-soothing.

Although children with ASD may not be distressed during the performance of repetitive behaviors, these behaviors can be impairing due to the time spent as well as the child's distress, noncompliance, and protest when repetitive behaviors are interrupted (Scahill et al. 2006). Some children with ASD perform repetitive behaviors in public places that stand out and contribute to social disability (Turner-Brown et al. 2011; Scahill et al. 2014).

In a sample of 272 children with ASD (age 4–17 years), we used principal components analysis to evaluate the symptom checklist on the Children's Yale-Brown Obsessive-Compulsive Scales for ASD (CYBOCS-ASD) (Scahill et al. 2014). The study sample consisted of participants in one of three clinical trials conducted by the Research Units on Pediatric Psychopharmacology (RUPP) Autism Network. The symptom checklist included 39 items, most of which were from the original list of compulsions on the CYBOCS. This measure was designed to assess severity of obsessions and compulsions in children with OCD (Scahill et al. 1997). When applied to the ASD sample, 15 checklist items were endorsed by less than 5 % of the sample (e.g., checking related to harm reduction, excessive cleaning, excessive list making, repetitive behavior to prevent harm, superstitious behavior) and were dropped from further analysis. As noted above, checking and other repetitive behavior to protect against harm and excessive cleaning are common in children with OCD – but were clearly uncommon in this sample of well-characterized children with ASD. The principal components analysis identified five categories: ritualistic behavior, ordering and arranging behavior, sameness and self-injurious behavior, and restricted interest (see Table 3.1 for examples). Although many children exhibited behaviors from more than one category, some behaviors were associated with cognitive ability. Children in the normal intelligence quotient (IQ) range were more likely to perform complex ritualistic behavior (Scahill et al. 2014). Consistent with other reports, children with intellectual disability were more likely to exhibit motor stereotypy and self-injurious behavior (Bishop et al. 2006).

Self-injurious behavior in children with ASD is a potentially serious problem that warrants separate discussion. In some children, self-injurious behavior is inadvertently reinforced by social reward such escape from a routine demand, obtaining a preferred object (a food or a toy) or obtaining caregiver attention. Alternatively, self-injurious behavior appears to be a repetitive, automatic behavior that is somehow self-reinforcing. These different types of self-injurious behavior (socially maintained vs automatic) may reflect of different underlying neural pathways (Oliver et al. 2012; Hagopian et al. 2015).

Given the wide range of cognitive functioning and language skills in children with ASD, distinguishing between the repetitive behaviors of ASD and behaviors that reflect the co-occurrence of OCD may be difficult (Bishop et al. 2013; Scahill et al.

Table 3.1 Product of principal component analysis[a] of CYBOCS-ASD checklist in 272 children with ASD

Ritualistic behavior	Sensory motor and arranging	Sameness and self-injurious behavior	Stereotypy	Restricted interest
Difficulty throwing things away	Lining up objects (toys, furniture)	Re-reading same book	Hand flapping, shaking fingers in front of eyes	Touching in patterns
Counting objects, repeating certain numbers	Echolalia	Insisting on routines (driving directions, morning routine)	Repeating routine activities (e.g., opening and closing doors)	Preoccupations (e.g., trains, specific videos, fans)
Checking locks, checking that objects are in the right place	Rocking, spinning, pacing	Head banging, biting own hand, hitting self	Object stereotypy (spinning object, shaking a pen or piece of string, etc.)	
Ritualized eating behavior (food prepared in specific way)	Repetitive water play (flushing and re-flushing toilet)	Masturbation, crotch grabbing		
Hair pulling, skin picking, nail biting				

[a]Principal component analysis was used to explore the *dimensionality* of the CYBOCS checklist

2014). Some children with ASD may be able to report why they perform repetitive behaviors; others may not. The inability to describe the purpose of the repetitive behavior is obvious for nonverbal children with ASD. Even children with language, however, may not be able to describe the link between an obsession (e.g., worry about harm) and the compulsion (complex touching behavior to reduce harm). Thus, clinicians may need to focus on observable behavior. Results of the meta-analysis, however, suggest that some children with ASD have a clinical picture that warrants a separate diagnosis of OCD (van Steensel et al. 2011). Lewin and colleagues (2011) compared OCD symptom picture in 35 children with high-functioning ASD and OCD to a group of 35 children with OCD (without ASD). In this study, the investigators used the original CYBOCS checklist and found some differences in symptom type and no difference in severity across the two groups. In the OCD plus ASD group, however, common OCD symptoms such as checking and washing were not endorsed.

In summary, some children with ASD present a clinical picture that warrants a separate diagnosis of OCD. The clinical picture of children with ASD accompanied by OCD appears similar to OCD in children without ASD. In clinical practice, therefore, the possible co-occurrence of OCD warrants careful consideration. The

Table 3.2 Repetitive behavior, obsessions, and preoccupations in ASD and OCD

Diagnosis	Behaviors	Obsessions/preoccupation	Impairment/distress
ASD	Flapping, rocking, flipping objects, watching the same video, lining up objects,	Fans, air conditioners; fireman and fire trucks, insistence on routines (turn right at the corner)	Wastes time, interferes with daily living and social interaction, hinders constructive activities, upsets if behavior is interrupted (drawn to do it)
OCD	Washing, checking, repetitive touching or repeating routine behavior to prevent harm, ordering and arranging, contamination worries	Contamination, harm to self or others, need for symmetry	Wastes time, interferes with daily living and social interaction, leads to avoidance. Unwanted thoughts repetitive behavior cause ↓ anxiety (has to do it)

12.5 % prevalence estimate of OCD in children with ASD is higher than the prevalence in the general pediatric population. If this estimate is accurate, it is clear that most children with ASD do not have OCD. Indeed, the repetitive behaviors for most children with ASD are not the same as the compulsions of OCD (see Table 3.2). Children with ASD may not be distressed about repetitive behavior. Indeed, protest and disruptive behavior may occur when the child is interrupted or blocked from performing the preferred repetitive behavior. Preoccupations with restricted interests in children with ASD are not the same as the nagging and unwanted obsessional thoughts in children with OCD.

6   Response to Selective Serotonin Reuptake Inhibitors

Alterations in serotonin neurotransmission have long been proposed as having a role in the pathophysiology of ASD. Medications such as selective serotonin reuptake inhibitors (SSRIs) are commonly used in children with ASD (Oswald and Sonenklar 2007; Coury et al. 2012; Romanelli et al. 2014). This frequent use of the SSRIs in treatment of children with ASD is due, at least in part, to the success of this medication class for the treatment of children with OCD (King et al. 2009). Findings from randomized clinical trials on the efficacy of the SSRIs for the treatment of repetitive behavior in ASD have been inconsistent. In adults with ASD, fluvoxamine (McDougle et al. 1996) and fluoxetine (Hollander et al. 2012) each showed superiority to placebo for reducing repetitive behavior. Hollander and colleagues conducted a placebo-controlled study of fluoxetine in 39 children and reported modest but statistically greater reductions in repetitive behaviors versus placebo (Hollander et al. 2005). In stark contrast, two large-scale randomized trials used the Children's Yale-Brown Obsessive-Compulsive Scales (CYBOCS-ASD) to measure repetitive behavior before and after treatment (Scahill et al. 2015b). In a sample of 149 children with ASD, liquid citalopram was no better than placebo (King et al. 2009). Similarly, in a sample of 158 children with ASD, an oral disintegrating formulation of fluoxetine (Neuropharm, clinicaltrials.gov 2011) was not superior to placebo for reducing repetitive behaviors. The seeming difference in response to SSRIs in adults with ASD compared to children with ASD is difficult to explain (Esbensen et al. 2009). The failure of SSRIs for reducing repetitive behavior in two separate, large-scale trials in children with ASD compared to the demonstrated benefit in children with OCD, however, implies differences in underlying neurobiology for the repetitive behavior in ASD versus OCD.

References

Alexander GE, DeLong MR, Strick PL (1986) Parallel organization of functionally segregated circuits linking basal ganglia and cortex. Annu Rev Neurosci 9:357–381

American Psychiatric Association (APA) (2000) Diagnostic and statistical manual of mental disorders-text revised (DSM-IV-TR), 4th edn. American Psychiatric Association (APA), Washington, DC

American Psychiatric Association (APA) (2013) Diagnostic and statistical manual of mental disorders-fifth edition (DSM 5). American Psychiatric Association (APA), Washington, DC

Arnott B, McConachie H, Meins E, Fernyhough C, Le Couteur A, Turner M, Parkinson K, Vittorini L, Leekam S (2009) The frequency of restricted and repetitive behaviours in 15 month-old typically developing infants. J Dev Behav Pediatr: JDBP 31(3):223–229

Banaschewski T, Brandeis D, Heinrich H, Albrecht B, Brunner E, Rothenberger A (2003) Association of ADHD and conduct disorder – brain electrical evidence for the existence of a distinct subtype. J Child Psychol Psychiatry 44(3):356–376

Baron-Cohen S (1989) Do autistic children have obsessions and compulsions? Br J Clin Psychol 28:193–200

Bearss K, Taylor CA, Aman MG, Whittemore R, Lecavalier L, Miller J, Pritchett J, Green B, Scahill L (2015) Using qualitative methods to guide scale development for anxiety in youth with autism spectrum disorder. Autism. Online ahead of print

Berridge KC, Aldridge JW, Houchard KR, Zhuang X (2005) Sequential superstereotypy of aninstinctive fixed action pattern in hyperdopaminergic mutant mice: a model of obsessive compulsive disorder and Tourette's. BMC Biol 3:4

Bishop SL, Richler J, Lord C (2006) Association between restricted and repetitive behaviors and nonverbal IQ in children with autism spectrum disorders. Child Neuropsychol: J Norm Abnorm Dev Child Adolesc 12(4–5):247–267

Bishop SL, Hus V, Duncan A, Huerta M, Gotham K, Pickles A, Kreiger A, Buja A, Lund S, Lord C (2013) Subcategories of restricted and repetitive behaviors in children with autism spectrum disorders. J Autism Dev Disord 43(6):1287–1297

Bodfish JW, Symons FJ, Parker D, Lewis MH (2000) Varieties of repetitive behavior in autism: comparisons to mental retardation. J Autism Dev Disord 30:237–243

Cipriani G, Vedovello M, Ulivi M, Nuti A, Lucetti C (2013) Repetitive and stereotypic phenomena and dementia. Am J Alzheimers Dis Other Demen 28(3):223–227

Coury DL, Anagnostou E, Manning-Courtney P, Reynolds A, Cole L, McCoy R, Whitaker A, Perrin JM (2012) Use of psychotropic medication in children and adolescents with autism spectrum disorders. Pediatrics 130(Suppl 2):S69–S76

de Wit S, Dickinson A (2009) Associative theories of goal-directed behaviour: a case for animal-human translational models. Psychol Res 73:463–476

Diniz JB, Rosario-Campos MC, Shavitt RG, Curi M, Hounie AG, Brotto SA, Miguel EC (2004) Impact of age at onset and duration of illness on the expression of comorbidities in obsessive-compulsive disorder. J Clin Psychiatry 65(1):22–27

Esbensen AJ, Seltzer MM, Lam KSL, Bodfish JW (2009) Age-related differences in restricted repetitive behaviors in autism spectrum disorders. J Autism Dev Disord 39:57–66

Gadow KD, DeVincent CJ, Pomeroy J (2006) ADHD symptom subtypes in children with pervasive developmental disorder. J Autism Dev Disord 36(2):271–283

Geller DA (2006) Obsessive-compulsive and spectrum disorders in children and adolescents. Psychiatr Clin North Am 29(2):353–370

Graybiel AM (2008) Habits, rituals, and the evaluative brain. Annu Rev Neurosci 31:359–387

Hagopian LP, Rooker G R, Zarcone JR (2015). Toward the identification of subtypes of self-injurious behavior maintained by automatic reinforcement. Journal of Applied Behavior Analysis, 48:523–543.

Hollander E, Phillips A, Chaplin W, Zagursky K, Novotny S, Wasserman S, Iyengar R (2005) A placebo controlled crossover trial of liquid fluoxetine on repetitive behaviors in childhood and adolescent autism. Neuropsychopharmacology 30(3):582–589

Hollander E, Soorya L, Chaplin W, Anagnostou E, Taylor BP, Ferretti CJ, Wasserman S, Swanson E, Settipani C (2012) A double-blind placebo-controlled trial of fluoxetine for repetitive behaviors and global severity in adult autism spectrum disorders. Am J Psychiatry 169(3):292–299

Honey E, McConachie H, Turner M, Rodgers J (2012a) Validation of the repetitive behaviour questionnaire for use with children with autism spectrum disorder. Res Autism Spectr Dis 6:355–362

Honey E, Rodgers J, McConachie H (2012b) Measurement of restricted and repetitive behaviour in children with autism spectrum disorder: selecting a questionnaire or interview. Res Autism Spectr Dis 6(2):757–776

John CE, McCracken CB, Haber SN (2010) Motivation on the Mediterranean: reward, compulsions and habit formation. Neurosci Biobehav Rev 34(1):2–6

Kerns CM, Kendall PC (2012) The presentation and classification of anxiety in autism spectrum disorder. Clin Psychol: Sci Pract 19(4):323–347

King BH, Hollander E, Sikich L, McCracken JT, Scahill L, Bregman JD, Donnelly CL, Anagnostou E, Dukes K, Sullivan L, Hirtz D, Wagner A, Ritz L, STAART Psychopharmacology Network (2009) Lack of efficacy of citalopram in children with autism spectrum disorders and high levels of repetitive behavior: citalopram ineffective in children with autism. Arch Gen Psychiatry 66(6):583–590

Lam KS, Aman MG (2007) The repetitive behavior scale–revised: independent validation in individuals with autism spectrum disorders. J Autism Dev Disord 37(5):855–866

Lam KSL, Bodfish JW, Piven J (2008) Evidence for three subtypes of repetitive behavior in autism that differ in familiality and association with other symptoms. J Child Psychol Psychiatry 49(11):1193–1200

Lecavalier L, Wood JJ, Halladay AK, Jones NE, Aman MG, Cook EH, Handen BL, King BH, Pearson DA, Hallett V, Sullivan KA, Grondhuis S, Bishop SL, Horrigan JP, Dawson G, Scahill L (2014) Measuring anxiety as a treatment endpoint in youth with autism spectrum disorder. J Autism Dev Disord 44(5):1128–1143

Leckman JF, Grice DE, Boardman J, Zhang H, Vitale A, Bondi C, Alsobrook J, Peterson BS, Cohen DJ, Rasmussen SA, Goodman WK, McDougle CJ, Pauls DL (1997) Symptoms of obsessive–compulsive disorder. Am J Psychiatry 154:911–917

Leckman JF, Peterson BS, King RA, Scahill L, Cohen DJ (2001) Phenomenology of tics and natural history of tic disorders. Adv Neurol 85:1–14

Leekam S, Tandos J, McConachie H, Meins E, Parkinson K, Wright C, Turner M, Arnott B, Vittorini L, Le Couteur A (2007) Repetitive behaviours in typically developing 2-year-olds. J Child Psychol Psychiatry 48(11):1131–1138

Lewin AB, Wood JJ, Gunderson S, Murphy TK, Storch EA (2011) Phenomenology of comorbid autism spectrum and obsessive-compulsive disorders among children. J Dev Phys Disabil 23:543–553

Lewis M, Kim SJ (2009) The pathophysiology of restricted repetitive behavior. J Neurodevelopmental Dis 1(2):114–132

Mataix-Cols D, do Rosario-Campos MC, Leckman JF (2005) A multidimensional model of obsessive–compulsive disorder. Am J Psychiatry 162:228–238

McDougle CJ, Kresch LE, Goodman WK, Naylor ST, Volkmar FR, Cohen DJ, Price LH (1995) A case-controlled study of repetitive thoughts and behavior in adults with autistic disorder and obsessive-compulsive disorder. Am J Psychiatry 152(5):772–777

McDougle CJ, Naylor ST, Cohen DJ, Volkmar FR, Heninger GR, Price LH (1996) A double-blind, placebo-controlled study of fluvoxamine in adults with autistic disorder. Arch Gen Psychiatry 53(11):1001–1008

Miguel EC, Leckman JF, Rauch S, do Rosario-Campos MC, Hounie AG, Mercadante MT, Chacon P, Pauls DL (2005) Obsessive–compulsive disorder phenotypes: implications for genetic studies. Mol Psychiatry 10:258–275

Mirenda P, Smith IM, Vaillancourt T, Georgiades S, Duku E, Szatmari P et al (2010) Validating the repetitive behavior scale-revised in young children with autism spectrum disorder. J Autism Dev Disord 40(12):1521–1530

Monzani B, Rijsdijk F, Harris J, Mataix-Cols D (2014) The structure of genetic and environmental risk factors for dimensional representations of DSM-5 obsessive-compulsive spectrum disorders. JAMA Psychiatry 71(2):182–189

Morrens M, Hulstijn W, Lewi PJ, De Hert M, Sabbe BG (2006) Stereotypy in schizophrenia. Schizophr Res 84:397–404

Moss J, Oliver C, Arron K, Burbidge C, Berg K (2009) The prevalence and phenomenology of repetitive behavior in genetic syndromes. J Autism Dev Dis 39:572–588

Nestadt G, Samuels JF, Riddle MA, Bienvenu OJ, Liang KY, Grados MA, Cullen B (2002) Obsessive-compulsive disorder: defining the phenotype. J Clin Psychiatry 63(Suppl 6):5–7

Neuropharm. Study of fluoxetine in autism (SOFIA). Available at: http://clinicaltrials.ov/ct2/show/NCT00515320. Accessed 23 Apr 2011

Oliver C, Petty J, Ruddick L, Bacarese-Hamilton M (2012) The association between repetitive, self-injurious and aggressive behavior in children with severe intellectual disability. J Autism Dev Dis 42:910–919

Oswald DP, Sonenklar NA (2007) Medication use among children with autism spectrum disorders. J Child Adolesc Psychopharmacol 17(3):348–355

Piacentini J (2008) Optimizing cognitive-behavioral therapy for childhood psychiatric disorders. J Am Acad Child Adolesc Psychiatry 47(5):481–482

Rauch SL, Jenike MA (1993) Neurobiological models of obsessive-compulsive disorder. Psychosomatics 34(1):20–32

Reiersen AM, Constantino JN, Volk HE, Todd RD (2007) Autistic traits in a population-based ADHD twin sample. J Child Psychol Psychiatry 48(5):464–472

Rettew DC, Swedo SE, Leonard HL, Lenane MC, Rapoport JL (1992) Obsessions and compulsions across time in 79 children and adolescents with obsessive-compulsive disorder. J Am Acad Child Adolesc Psychiatry 31(6):1050–1056

Romanelli RJ, Wu FM, Gamba R, Mojtabai R, Segal JB (2014) Behavioral therapy and serotonin reuptake inhibitor pharmacotherapy in the treatment of obsessive-compulsive disorder: a systematic review and meta-analysis of head-to-head randomized controlled trials. Depression Anxiety 31(8):641–652

Rosario-Campos MC, Miguel EC, Quatrano S, Chacon P, Ferrao Y, Findley D, Katsovich L, Scahill L, King RA, Woody SR, Tolin D, Hollander E, Kano Y, Leckman JF (2006) The dimensional Yale-Brown obsessive-compulsive scale (DY-BOCS): an instrument for assessing obsessive-compulsive symptom dimensions. J Mol Psychiatry 11(5):495–504

Scahill L, Riddle MA, McSwiggin-Hardin M, Ort SI, King RA, Goodman WK, Cicchetti D, Leckman JF (1997) Children's Yale-Brown obsessive compulsive scale: reliability and validity. J Am Acad Child Adolesc Psychiatry 36(6):844–852

Scahill L, Kano Y, King RA, Carlson A, Peller A, LeBrun U, do Rosario-Campos MC, Leckman JF (2003) Influence of age and tic disorders on obsessive-compulsive disorder in a pediatric sample. J Child Adolesc Psychopharmacol 13(Suppl 1):S7–S17

Scahill L, McDougle CJ, Williams SK, Dimitropoulos A, Aman MG, McCracken JT, Tierney E, Arnold LE, Cronin P, Grados M, Ghuman J, Koenig K, Lam KS, McGough J, Posey DJ, Ritz L, Swiezy NB, Vitiello B, Research Units on Pediatric Psychopharmacology Autism Network (2006) The Children's Yale-Brown obsessive compulsive scales modified for pervasive developmental disorders. J Am Acad Child Adolesc Psychiatry 45(9):1114–1123

Scahill L, Dimitropoulos A, McDougle CJ, Aman MG, Feurer ID, McCracken JT, Tierney E, Pu J, White S, Lecavalier L, Hallett V, Bearss K, King B, Arnold LE, Vitiello B (2014) Children's Yale-Brown obsessive compulsive scale in autism spectrum disorder: component structure of symptom checklist and distribution of severity scales. J Am Acad Child Adolesc Psychiatry 53(1):97–107

Scahill L, Aman MG, Lecavalier L, Halladay AK, Bishop SL, Bodfish JW, Grondhuis S, Jones N, Horrigan JP, Cook EH, Handen BL, King BH, Pearson DA, McCracken JT, Sullivan KA, Dawson G (2015a) Measuring repetitive behaviors as a treatment endpoint in youth with autism spectrum disorder. Autism 19(1):38–52

Scahill L, Sukhodolsky DG, Anderberg E, Dimitropoulos A, Dziura J, Aman MG, McCracken J, Tierney E, Hallett V, Katz K, Vitiello B, McDougle C (2015b) Sensitivity of the modified children's Yale-Brown obsessive compulsive scale to detect change: results from two multi-site trials. Autism 19(1):38–52

Simonoff E, Pickles A, Charman T, Chandler S, Loucas T, Baird G (2008) Psychiatric disorders in children with autism spectrum disorders: prevalence, comorbidity, and associated factors in a population-derived sample. J Am Acad Child Adolesc Psychiatry 47(8):921–929

Turner M (1999) Annotation: repetitive behaviour in autism: a review of psychological research. J Child Psychol Psychiatry 40(6):839–849

Turner-Brown LM, Lam KSL, Holtzclaw TN, Dichter GS, Bodfish JW (2011) Phenomenology and measurement of circumscribed interests in autism spectrum disorders. Autism 15(4):437–456

van Steensel FJ, Bögels SM, Perrin S (2011) Anxiety disorders in children and adolescents with autistic spectrum disorders: a meta-analysis. Clin Child Fam Psychol Rev 14(3):302–317

World Health Organization (WHO) (2007) The ICD-10 classification of mental and behavioural disorders: diagnostic criteria. WHO, Geneva

Schizophrenia Spectrum Disorders and Autism Spectrum Disorder

4

Katharine Chisholm, Ashleigh Lin, and Marco Armando

1 Introduction

Schizophrenia spectrum disorders (SSD) and autism spectrum disorder (ASD) are currently conceptualised as separate illnesses. SSD, as defined by the DSM-5, include schizophrenia, other psychotic disorders, and schizotypal personality disorder. This group of disorders involves delusions, hallucinations, disorganised thinking, disorganised behaviour, and negative symptoms. Definitions of ASD and SSD have undergone many revisions. Bleuler (1950) believed that autism was a central feature of schizophrenia, whilst others viewed it as the childhood onset of the disorder (Bender 1947). In fact, the term autism was used interchangeably with schizophrenia until the 1970s, when Rutter (1972) and Kolvin (1971) proposed that they were distinct disorders. The nosologic separation between ASD and SSD may initially appear justified given the distinct differences in age of onset and many differences in presentation. Yet, despite apparent differences, SSD and ASD share multiple phenotypic similarities and risk factors (Hamlyn et al. 2013; Spek and Wouters 2010), have both been conceptualised as neurodevelopmental rather than neurodegenerative disorders (Goldstein et al. 2002), and have been reported to

K. Chisholm (✉)
School of Psychology, University of Birmingham, Birmingham, UK
e-mail: K.e.chisholm.1@bham.ac.uk

A. Lin
Telethon Kids Institute, The University of Western Australia, Perth, Australia
e-mail: Ashleigh.Lin@telethonkids.org.au

M. Armando
Child and Adolescence Neuropsychiatry Unit, Department of Neuroscience,
I.R.C.C.S. Bambino Gesù Children's Hospital, Rome, Italy

Office Médico-Pédagogique Research Unit, Department of Psychiatry, University of Geneva
School of Medicine, Geneva, Switzerland
e-mail: marco.armando@opbg.net

© Springer International Publishing Switzerland 2016   51
L. Mazzone, B. Vitiello (eds.), *Psychiatric Symptoms and Comorbidities in
Autism Spectrum Disorder*, DOI 10.1007/978-3-319-29695-1_4

co-occur at elevated rates (Mouridsen et al. 2008a, b; Rapoport et al. 2009; Solomon et al. 2011; Stahlberg et al. 2004). Systematic research on their co-occurrence has been limited, although emerging genetic and neuroanatomical evidence has led to increasing recognition of the overlap between the conditions (Carroll and Owen 2009; Cheung et al. 2010).

In this chapter, we describe prevalence rates of overlap between the ASD and SSD at a clinical and trait level and discuss difficulties in the diagnosis and evaluation of the disorders. We then discuss genetic and neurobiological evidence, highlighting similarities and areas of distinction between the disorders. Finally, we briefly present treatment options, including non-medical and novel treatment strategies as well as pharmacological interventions.

2 Prevalence

Although there have been reports that SSD and ASD do not co-occur at elevated rates (Volkmar and Cohen 1991), the majority of research suggests that the disorders co-occur at a higher rate than would be expected in the general population. As ASD and SSD both occur in around 1 % of the population (Brugha et al. 2011; Kendler et al. 1996; Baio 2012; van Os et al. 2001), studies with fewer than 100 participants are unlikely to be truly representative. We have identified 14 papers that showed overlapping prevalence of ASD and SSD published since 2004 (Table 4.1). Of these, nine investigate rates of SSD in ASD populations (Bakken et al. 2010; Billstedt et al. 2005; Eaves and Ho 2008; Hofvander et al. 2009; Joshi et al. 2010; Lugnegard et al. 2011; Mouridsen et al. 2008a, b; Stahlberg et al. 2004), and five examined rates of ASD in those diagnosed with SSD (Davidson et al. 2014; Hallerback et al. 2012; Solomon et al. 2011; Sporn et al. 2004; Waris et al. 2013). Only six had samples >100 (Billstedt et al. 2005; Davidson et al. 2014; Hofvander et al. 2009; Joshi et al. 2010; Mouridsen et al. 2008a, b). These papers found a mean incidence of 12.8 % of SSD in ASD populations, with only one study reporting on ASD in SSD with a sample of over 100 (Davidson et al. 2014) and finding an incidence rate of 3.6 %. Large population studies are needed to ascertain true diagnostic comorbidities in ASD and SSD.

3 Phenomenology and Clinical Issues

As well as the high prevalence of comorbidity between ASD and SSD, there is also an overlap in terms of symptoms, at both clinical (Waris et al. 2013) and subclinical (Bevan Jones et al. 2012) levels. Moreover, neurodevelopmental abnormalities frequently found in children with ASD, such as a delay in motor development and impaired receptive language, and relationship and adjustment difficulties are frequently found as prodromal features of SSD (Owen et al. 2011). Likewise, childhood deficits documented in those who later develop SSD mimic ASD traits (Dickson et al. 2011). Whilst in neurotypical adults with well-described

Table 4.1   Rates of co-occurrence between ASD and SSD

Authors	n	% co-occurrence
SSD in ASD populations		
Eaves and Ho (2008)	48 young adults with ASD	0 %
Lugnegard et al. (2011)	54 young adults with Asperger syndrome	3.7 %
Mouridsen et al. (2008a, b)	118 individuals diagnosed as children with infantile autism	6.6 %
Billstedt et al. (2005)	120 individuals with autism diagnosed in childhood	7 %
Hofvander et al. (2009)	122 adults with normal intelligence ASD	12 %
Stahlberg et al. (2004)	129 adults diagnosed with ASD	14.8 %
Joshi et al. (2010)	217 children and adolescents meeting diagnostic criteria for an ASD	20 %
Bakken et al. (2010)	62 adults with autism and intellectual disability	25.1 %
Mouridsen et al. (2008a, b)	89 individuals with atypical autism	34.8 %
ASD in SSD populations		
Davidson et al. (2014)	197 adults attending an early intervention in psychosis service	3.6 %
Sporn et al. (2004)	75 children with COS	3.9 %
Solomon et al. (2011)	16 individuals with first episode of psychosis	19 %
Waris et al. (2013)	18 adolescents with early-onset schizophrenia	44 %
Hallerback et al. (2012)	46 adults with a diagnoses of schizophrenic psychotic disorders	50–60 %

symptoms differentiating between psychotic and autistic symptoms is not particularly challenging, diagnostic difficulties are more common in the early phase of these disorders, when symptoms are less clear cut, or in individuals who lack the receptive or expressive language skills to describe their symptoms (Dossetor 2007). Hallucinatory experiences, for example, are often reported in individuals with ASD, although differentiating between an external voice and an internal dialogue may be difficult. In this regard, sensory abnormalities are reported in as many as 90 % of children with ASD and can be misinterpreted as hallucinations (Leekam et al. 2007). Conversely, some symptoms, which are core feature of ASD, are frequently seen and often misinterpreted in individuals with SSD. For example, a deficit in emotion recognition, leading to misinterpretations of the actions of others as paranoid delusions, is a core feature of ASD and also common in SSD (Kaland et al. 2008).

Given the arbitrary nature of diagnostic thresholds and the heterogeneity of presentations of individuals with ASD and SSD, it is important to consider the co-occurrence at the trait level. A descriptive overlap exists in the traits that make up the diagnostic criteria for ASD and SSD. Both disorders include deficits in social interaction and communication as primary symptoms; the lack of emotional reciprocity in ASD can be compared to blunted affect (a lack of emotional response) in

SSD; the delay or lack of speech development in ASD parallels alogia (poverty of speech) in SSD; and catatonic features are observed in both diagnoses. It is perhaps unsurprising that much research has found co-occurrence of traits such as these (e.g. Brüne 2005; Spek and Wouters 2010). Similarities are also found in traits that relate to, but are not part of, the diagnostic criteria. Theory of mind and mentalising impairments are hypothesised to be central to both disorders (Baron-Cohen et al. 1985; Bora et al. 2009; Brüne 2005; Chung et al. 2013). Similarly, Eack et al. (2013) report that those with ASD and SSD experience similar deficits in their neurocognitive and social cognitive functioning.

Conversely, other authors report traits that do differentiate between the disorders. Intellectual disability, for example, is more common in ASD than SSD (Baio 2010; Cooper 1997; Morgan and Jorm 2008). Although both disorders show a higher male to female ratio in individuals diagnosed, the male-female ratio appears to be considerably higher in ASD than SSD (Ochoa et al. 2012; Wing 1981b). Level of communication deficits may also differentiate between ASD and SSD. In a study comparing individuals at risk for psychosis, those with a first episode of psychosis, individuals with autism, and healthy controls, Solomon and colleagues (2011) found that 20 % of those in the high risk or first-episode psychosis groups met diagnostic criteria for ASD as assessed by parental report. However, there were a number of traits which distinguished between the different diagnostic categories. Atypical developmental trajectories in communication and social behaviours, as well as structural and pragmatic language, were found to a much greater extent in the ASD group compared to the SSD and control groups. Similarly, when comparing individuals with ASD and SSD, Spek and Wouters (2010) demonstrated that individuals with ASD reported more impairment with social skills, attention switching, and communication than those with SSD.

There is also longitudinal evidence for an overlap between ASD and SSD at the trait level. Evidence from two large cohort studies has confirmed that the presence of psychotic experiences at age 12 is associated with ASD traits earlier in life (Bevan Jones et al. 2012; Sullivan et al. 2013). Similarly, meta-analysis has recently confirmed that childhood deficits documented in those who later develop SSD mimic ASD traits (Dickson et al. 2011). Whether these traits reflect aspects of ASD which were undiagnosed or did not reach clinical significance or instead reflect the status of SSD as a neurodevelopmental disorder remains to be determined.

Other research suggests, however, that ASD traits may not be predictive of the development of SSD. A study from Vorstman and colleagues (2013) investigated childhood ASD traits in 78 patients with 22q11.2 deletion syndrome, 36 of whom had developed psychotic disorder. High levels of ASD traits were reported to have occurred during childhood in their population, but were not predictive of the development of SSD. Higher rates of ASD traits had a stronger association with the non-psychotic individuals with the deletion, suggesting that, in the case of 22q11.2 deletion syndrome, the disorders share a genetic vulnerability but are distinct in their expression of this vulnerability.

4   Peculiar Features of the Disorder in Comorbidity with ASD

As can be seen in the section above, there are many shared traits or symptoms between those diagnosed with ASD and those diagnosed with SSD. Despite this, often symptoms can still be distinctive. For example, in ASD misinterpretations of other's behaviours/emotions, which lead to delusions, are mostly caused by a lack of social cognition (Blackshaw et al. 2001). On the other hand, in people with SSD, the process that leads to delusion formation is mostly driven by affective dysregulation (Smeets et al. 2012), rather than a deficit in social cognition. Thus, whilst it can be difficult to differentiate between individuals with ASD and SSD by focusing on clinical presentation of the delusional symptom alone, a clearer differentiation can be found at a phenomenological level. These differences in phenomenological characterisation of the delusion have relevant consequences in the choice of and response to treatments.

Beyond the peculiar features of psychotic symptoms in ASD and SSD, what is interesting to note is that, among individuals with from SSD, some are characterised by an evident autistic phenotype, whilst positive psychotic symptoms are less prominent (King and Lord 2011). Retrospective research has identified two subgroups within SSD populations: a larger group with relatively little behavioural impairment throughout childhood and a smaller group which displays early behavioural abnormalities (Corcoran et al. 2003; Rossi et al. 2000). This latter subgroup of patients can be characterised by difficulties in the metacognitive domain, emotion processing, and motor abnormalities (Cheung et al. 2010) as well as an earlier onset of SSD and a more chronic course of illness (Myin-Germeys and van Os 2007; Rossi et al. 2000). At the same time, this subgroup usually shows a prevalence of negative symptoms and obtains high scores on the Autism Diagnostic Observation Schedule (ADOS; Bastiaansen et al. 2011), leading some to suggest they may be a potential subgroup with a stronger association to ASD (Konstantareas and Hewitt 2001).

5   Diagnosis and Evaluation: Assessment Tools

Anecdotally, the diagnosis of ASD in SSD (and vice versa) poses problems. There are currently no assessment tools for differentiating ASD and SSD despite their common co-occurrence, and diagnosis is usually made via clinical interview. Unless an individual with SSD has been given a diagnosis with ASD as a child, the diagnosis of ASD is clinically challenging. For example, the clinician must differentiate negative symptoms from stable traits of ASD. Researchers have investigated ASD in populations with SSD and first-episode psychosis and individuals at ultra-high risk (UHR) for psychosis (the criteria for which are based on a combination of state and trait risk factors; the most common of these are attenuated positive psychotic symptoms below the threshold for a diagnosis of frank psychosis; Yung et al. 1996). Some researchers have employed lengthy diagnostic interviews such as the Diagnostic Interview for Social and Communication Disorders (DISCO; Wing 2006) to diagnose ASD in populations with SSD (Waris et al. 2013; Hallerback et al. 2012). Others have used the Social Communication Questionnaire (Rutter et al. 2003), which is based on the Autism Diagnostic Observation Schedule (ADOS), to approximate a diagnosis of ASD (Soloman et al. 2011; Sprong et al. 2008). ASD screening tools have also been used for this purpose (Davidson et al. 2014; Sporn et al. 2004), such as the Autism Screening Questionnaire (Berument et al. 1999) or Autism Spectrum Disorder in Adults Screening Questionnaire (Nylander and Gillberg 2001). However, these instruments may lack validity in a person help-seeking for psychological distress, and differentiating state and trait symptoms is challenging. Indeed, if an individual is floridly psychotic or psychologically very unwell, completing these measures may not be possible. Thus the comorbid diagnosis of ASD in SSD is best conducted after symptom stabilisation, with primary goal of diagnosis to be how therapy (particularly psychological therapy) might be best delivered.

The diagnosis of SSD in a person with ASD can be even more difficult. No assessment tools have been developed that account for many of the core features of ASD, in particular deficits in communication. Establishing the functional impact of psychosis is also a challenging task since individuals with ASD may to already have deficits in everyday functioning, especially within the social domain. In verbal individuals with ASD, semi-structured interviews, such as the Positive and Negative Symptom Scale (PANSS, Kay et al. 1987), may be useful for the determination of positive symptomology. Scales used to assess the UHR state may also be valuable, such as the Comprehensive Assessment of the At-Risk Mental State (CAARMS; Yung et al. 2005) or the Structured Interview for Prodromal Symptoms (SIPS; McGlashan et al. 2001). The advantage of these assessments is that subthreshold symptoms are captured. If the individual does meet the UHR criteria, it is up to the clinician to make the judgement on whether these symptoms represent the prodrome of a psychotic disorder or whether they are more stably related to the individual's ASD. All of these tools can be used to assess negative and disorganised symptoms in people with ASD, although determining if these types of symptoms are related to psychosis and require treatment or are state traits of ASD is more complex. In summary, we suggest that the diagnosing psychotic symptoms in individuals with ASD should be done by a multidisciplinary team via clinical interview and using the validated measures where possible. There is a clear need to develop improved means of diagnosis of psychosis in individuals with ASD.

6 Neurobiological Bases and Genetic Overlap

6.1 Genetic Risk Factors

ASD and SSD rates of heritability are both estimated to be high at around 50–80 % (Cardno and Gottesman 2000; Freitag 2006; Sandin et al. 2014). What is particularly interesting is the fact that, as well as showing high levels of heritability within each disorder, there is evidence of relatively high levels of heritability between the disorders (Daniels et al. 2008; Larsson et al. 2005; Sporn et al. 2004; Sullivan et al. 2012).

This is consistent with studies investigating copy number variants (CNVs; variations of DNA sequence in the genome) in SSD and ASD. Particular CNVs are implicated in both ASD and SSD, and specific rare alleles have been found to occur in both disorders (Lionel et al. 2013; McCarthy et al. 2009; Moreno-De-Luca et al. 2010; Weiss et al. 2008). The high number of shared CNV deletions and duplications, including NRXN1, CNTNAP2, 22q11.2, 1q21.1, and 15q13.3, led Carroll and Owens (2009) to conclude in their review that genetic evidence challenges the assumption that ASD and SSD are completely unrelated disorders.

A particularly compelling example of overlapping genetic vulnerability comes from the high rates of ASD and SSD seen in individuals with 22q11.2 deletion syndrome. In the largest study to date, investigators examined psychiatric morbidity in 1,402 individuals with the syndrome (Schneider et al. 2014). SSD were found in 1.97 % of children aged 6–12, 10.12 % of adolescents aged 13–17, 23.53 % of emerging adults aged 18–25, 41.33 % of young adults aged 26–35, and 41.73 % of mature adults aged 36 or above. Similarly high rates of ASD were also found, with rates varying across the life span of 12.77 % for children, to 26.54 % for adolescents, and to 16.10 % for adults.

There is also evidence of genetic differentiation between the disorders. Whilst CNVs appear to be enriched in individuals with ASD and SSD, common risk alleles have not generally been found to be shared between the disorders. Using genome-wide genotype data from the Cross-Disorder Group of the Psychiatric Genomics Consortium (2013), only a low genetic correlation was found between ASD and SSD. This suggests that common risk variants may play a limited role in ASD when compared to SSD, particularly when considering the lack of confirmed genome-wide association study results in ASD (Devlin et al. 2011).

6.2 Neurobiological Risk Factors

Neuroimaging evidence presents a similar picture to phenomenological and genetic risk factor research, with many similarities apparent between the disorders, but also some differences. In terms of similarities, both individuals with ASD and those with SSD have been found via meta-analysis to show reduced grey matter volume in limbic-striato-thalamic circuitry, predominantly on the right, including the insula, posterior cingulate, and parahippocampal gyrus (Cheung et al. 2010).

Reduced fractional anisotropy values (reflecting altered white matter integrity) have also been found in both disorders (Mueller et al. 2012). In ASD, implicated areas include the corpus callosum, the right corticospinal tract, the internal capsule, the left and right pedunculi cerebri, and the cingulate gyrus (Bloemen et al. 2010; Brito et al. 2009). Within SSD, implicated areas are the left frontal deep white matter including the frontal lobe, thalamus, and cingulate gyrus and the left temporal deep white matter including the frontal lobe, insula, hippocampus-amygdala complex, and temporal and occipital lobes (Ellison-Wright and Bullmore 2009).

Functional imaging analyses have focused on social cognition as a primary feature of both disorders. A meta-analysis has shown that brain regions thought to be part of a social cognition network show hypoactivation in both ASD and SSD in response to social stimuli, most consistently seen in the medial prefrontal cortex and superior temporal sulcus (Sugranyes et al. 2011). Similarly, a review from Abdi and Sharma (2004) found reductions in blood flow to the fusiform gyrus and abnormal amygdala activation during emotional perception tasks in both ASD and SSD.

Neurochemical abnormalities such as dopamine disruption have also been observed in both disorders (Cartier et al. 2015; Hérault et al. 1993; Muck-Seler et al. 2004; Stone et al. 2007). Within SSD dopamine disruption has been identified as a central feature of the disorder (Howes and Kapur 2009; Winton-Brown et al. 2014). Research into the dopamine system in ASD is more limited. In a study which compared eight adults with Asperger syndrome to five healthy controls using positron emission tomography (PET), Nieminen-von Wendt et al. (2004) found increased FDOPA influx (Ki) values in the striatum of the ASD group. Similarly, in another PET study which compared 20 individuals with ASD with control participants, an over-functioning of dopaminergic systems in the orbitofrontal cortex was suggested by a higher level of dopamine transporter bindings in the ASD group when compared to controls (Nakamura et al. 2010).

There are also potential areas of distinction between the disorders. These include increased cerebral ventricle volume and a reduction in overall brain volume found in individuals with SSD but not ASD (Shenton et al. 2001; Toal et al. 2009), as well as decreased white matter integrity, again found in individuals diagnosed with SSD but not ASD (Davis et al. 2003; Hao et al. 2006; Toal et al. 2009). A meta-analysis from Cheung et al. (2010), which aimed to quantify structural similarities between ASD and SSD, found that abnormalities in the right and left superior and medial frontal gyrus, right and left cingulate, left insula, caudate, temporal gyrus, and amygdala were specific to SSD and abnormalities in the left putamen appeared specific to ASD.

Other research, particularly studies investigating social deficits, has found opposing patterns of activation during functional magnetic resonance imaging (fMRI). A recent study from Ciaramidaro et al. (2014), which directly compared individuals with ASD and SSD on different types of intentionality, found that activation between the right posterior superior temporal sulcus and the ventral medial prefrontal cortex was abnormal in both groups, with an increased connectivity found in those with SSD and a decreased connectivity in those with ASD. The increased connectivity in SSD was found during the control condition ('physical intentionality', e.g. a balloon is blown by a gust of wind), and the decreased connectivity in ASD was found during the experimental intention condition. The authors argue that this is consistent with the hypo-hyper-intentionality hypothesis (Abu-Akel and Bailey 2000; Crespi and Badcock 2008) that individuals with SSD over-attribute intentions to others and physical events, whereas those with ASD often fail to attribute intentions to others. This hypothesis parallels evidence from EEG studies which find reduced Mu suppression (used as marker for mirror neuron activity) in ASD participants taking part in socio-emotional tasks (Oberman et al. 2005) and increased Mu suppression in those with SSD (McCormick et al. 2012).

A particularly interesting investigation of brain anatomy in individuals with ASD compared to those with comorbid ASD and SSD found that the primary differences in those with comorbid ASD and SSD (compared to those with ASD alone) related to reductions in grey matter in the right insular cortex, the cerebellum, the fusiform gyrus and the lingual gyri (Toal et al. 2009). Toal et al. (2009) note that their participants with comorbid ASD and SSD did not display the same changes usually found in populations who have developed SSD such as an increased volume of cerebral ventricles with a reduction in total brain volume (Shenton et al. 2001). They suggest that their comorbid population appear to share more anatomical similarities with individuals in UHR for psychosis groups rather than those with frank SSD and points out that the cerebellum and fusiform gyrus (which showed reductions in their comorbid population) have been implicated in UHR individuals (alongside left parahippocampal gyrus and the orbitofrontal and cingulate cortex, e.g. Job et al. 2005; Pantelis et al. 2003). Toal et al. suggest that these anatomical differences may hint that, for some individuals, ASD represent a different pathway into SSD.

7 Treatment

Whilst there is a robust literature on pharmacological and psychosocial treatments for ASD and SSD as separate disorders, there is a strong lack of evidence on the treatment of psychotic symptoms and SSD in comorbidity with ASD (Na Young and Findling 2015; Starling and Dossetor 2009). There is an established evidence base for early intervention in psychosis (Hollis 2013; Marshall and Rathbone 2011), which includes symptom-targeted interventions, low starting doses of atypical antipsychotics, psychoeducation for patients and families, other psychosocial interventions as needed, and assertive community treatment. Very limited data exist on the treatment of SSD in ASD, and to the best of our knowledge, no randomised controlled trials have been conducted to date.

7.1 Pharmacological Interventions

Antipsychotic drugs (APD) have had a long association with ASD (Cohen et al. 1978). Nevertheless, most of the studies are focused on the effectiveness of APD for the treatment of behavioural disorders in ASD. In this regard, the Research Units on Pediatric Psychopharmacology (RUPP) study (Arnold et al. 2003, 2005) showed their efficacy for treating disruptive behaviour in ASD (tantrums, aggression, and hyperactivity). However, a rapid return of disruptive and aggressive behaviour after discontinuation emerged. Second-generation antipsychotics (SGAs) in general (particularly risperidone and aripiprazole) appear to be more effective in controlling positive and disorganised symptoms (Ching and Pringsheim 2012; Na Young and Findling 2015). The side effects such as metabolic adverse events, including weight gain and dyslipidaemia, appear to be more common than in SSD without ASD (Arnold et al. 2005; Ching and Pringsheim 2012; Na Young and Findling 2015).

Overall, efficacy and tolerability of APD in patients with ASD and psychotic symptoms are less favourable than in patients with SSD alone (Ameis et al. 2013).

7.2   Non-medical Treatments

Similarly, limited data exist for non-medical treatment of psychotic symptoms in ASD. Psychosocial interventions are now recognised as important components of a comprehensive therapeutic approach in schizophrenia, improving outcomes, reducing negative symptoms, and increasing functional recovery. Moreover, pharmacological treatment alone has limited efficacy on negative symptoms and functional recovery (Hollis 2003). Consequently, there is a growing interest in psychosocial interventions, which are now recognised as an important component of a comprehensive therapeutic approach in schizophrenia (Armando et al. 2015). Indeed, there are relatively large numbers of randomised studies on the efficacy of psychosocial interventions such as cognitive-behavioural therapy, cognitive remediation, psychoeducation, and family intervention (Morrison et al. 2012; Puig et al. 2014; Wykes and Reeder 2005), and several systematic reviews have been conducted on this topic (Pilling et al. 2002; Tarrier et al. 2002). Nevertheless, there is a distinct lack of evidence regarding the efficacy of psychosocial interventions for psychotic symptoms in ASD. To date, no randomised controlled trial, systematic review, or meta-analysis has been conducted on this topic.

7.3   Novel Treatment Strategies

The relative success of APD in treating positive symptoms in SSD is limited by their lack of efficacy for negative and cognitive symptoms, which often determine the level of functional impairment. In addition, whilst SGAs produce fewer motor side effects, safety and tolerability concerns about metabolic syndrome have emerged. Consequently, there is an urgent need for more effective and better-tolerated APD and to identify new molecular targets. Following this evidence, a variety of new experimental pharmacological approaches have emerged in SSD recently, including molecules acting on targets other than the dopamine D2 receptor. In this context, future drug development strategies can fall into three categories: (1) improvement of precedent mechanisms of action to provide drugs of comparable or superior efficacy and side effect profiles to existing APD, (2) development of non-D2 mechanism APD, and (3) development of interventions as adjuncts to APD to augment efficacy by targeting specific symptom dimensions of SSD (Miyamoto et al. 2012). In this regard, newer agents, including glutamatergic agents, oxytocin, tolcapone, and entacapone, appear promising albeit with mixed results (Apud and Weinberger 2007; Gupta et al. 2011; Na Young and Findling 2015). Nevertheless, none of these novel treatment strategies, as well as previous well-consolidated pharmacological and non-pharmacological intervention for SSD, have been tested, validated, and replicated for psychotic symptoms in ASD. To date only few open-label studies exist on the efficacy of those interventions in this group of patients.

8 Discussion and Future Directions

It is becoming increasingly evident that it is necessary to prospectively investigate the co-occurrence of, and commonalities between, SSD and ASD at the trait level using multifactorial data from large samples. Undiagnosed co-occurring disorders may result in individuals not receiving appropriate services, benefits, or treatment, and given the similarities between disorders, misdiagnosis is possible (Davidson et al. 2014; Wing 1981a). There is clearly a need for the development of appropriate diagnostic tools to differentiate between ASD and SSD and for research investigating optimal pharmacological treatments of patients presenting with both disorders. It is important that future research accounts for the heterogeneity of both disorders and examines evidence on multiple levels to identify endophenotypic markers, as well as taking the dimensional nature of the disorders into consideration. Together, these approaches can provide an important conceptual framework for understanding the association between ASD and SSD. This in turn may lead towards the development of a fundamental understanding of the two disorders.

References

Abdi Z, Sharma T (2004) Social cognition and its neural correlates in schizophrenia and autism. CNS Spectr 9:335–343

Abu-Akel A, Bailey AL (2000) Letter. Psychol Med 30(03):735–738

Ameis SH, Corbett-Dick P, Cole L, Correll CU (2013) Decision making and antipsychotic medication treatment for youth with autism spectrum disorders: applying guidelines in the real world. J Clin Psychiatry 74(10):1022–1024

Apud JA, Weinberger DR (2007) Treatment of cognitive deficits associated with schizophrenia. CNS Drugs 21(7):535–557

Armando M, Pontillo M, Vicari S (2015) Psychosocial interventions for very early and early-onset schizophrenia: a review of treatment efficacy. Curr Opin Psychiatry 28:312–323

Arnold LE, Vitiello B, McDougle C et al (2003) Parent defined target symptoms respond to risperidone in RUPP autism study: customer approach to clinical trials. J Am Acad Child Adolesc Psychiatry 42:1143–1450

Arnold LE, Vitiello B, McDougle C et al (2005) Risperidone treatment of autistic disorder: longer-term benefits and blinded discontinuation after 6 months. Am J Psychiatry 162(7):1361–1369

Baio J (2010) Prevalence of autism spectrum disorder among children aged 8 years – autism and developmental disabilities monitoring network, 11 Sites, United States. Centers for Disease Control and Prevention

Baio J (2012) Prevalence of autism spectrum disorders: autism and developmental disabilities monitoring network, 14 sites, United States, 2008. Morbidity and mortality weekly report. Surveillance Summaries. Vol. 61(3). Centers for Disease Control and Prevention

Bakken TL, Helverschou SB, Eilertsen DE, Heggelund T, Myrbakk E, Martinsen H (2010) Psychiatric disorders in adolescents and adults with autism and intellectual disability: a representative study in one county in Norway. Res Dev Disabil 31(6):1669–1677

Baron-Cohen S, Leslie AM, Frith U (1985) Does the autistic child have a "theory of mind"? Cognition 21(1):37–46

Bastiaansen JA, Meffert H, Hein S, Huizinga P, Ketelaars C, Pijnenborg M, de Bildt A (2011) Diagnosing autism spectrum disorders in adults: the use of Autism Diagnostic Observation Schedule (ADOS) module 4. J Autism Dev Disord 41(9):1256–1266

Bender L (1947) Childhood schizophrenia. Am J Orthopsychiatry 17(1):40–56

Berument SK, Rutter M, Lord C, Pickles A, Bailey A (1999) Autism screening questionnaire: diagnostic validity. Br J Psychiatry 175(5):444–451

Bevan Jones R, Thapar A, Lewis G, Zammit S (2012) The association between early autistic traits and psychotic experiences in adolescence. Schizophr Res 135:164–169

Billstedt E, Gillberg C, Gillberg C (2005) Autism after adolescence: population-based 13-to 22-year follow-up study of 120 individuals with autism diagnosed in childhood. J Autism Dev Disord 35(3):351–360

Blackshaw AJ, Kinderman P, Hare DJ, Hatton C (2001) Theory of mind, causal attribution and paranoia in Asperger syndrome. Autism 5(2):147–163

Bleuler E (1950) Dementia Praecox or the Group of Schizophrenias, 1911 (English translation: J. Zinkin). International Universities Press, New York

Bloemen OJ, Deeley Q, Sundram F, Daly EM, Barker GJ, Jones DK, Murphy KC (2010) White matter integrity in Asperger syndrome: a preliminary diffusion tensor magnetic resonance imaging study in adults. Autism Res 3(5):203–213

Bora E, Yucel M, Pantelis C (2009) Theory of mind impairment in schizophrenia: meta-analysis. Schizophr Res 109(1):1–9

Brito AR, Vasconcelos MM, Domingues RC, da Cruz Jr H, Celso L, Rodrigues LDS, Calçada CABP (2009) Diffusion tensor imaging findings in school-aged autistic children. J Neuroimaging 19(4):337–343

Brugha TS, McManus S, Bankart J, Scott F, Purdon S, Smith J, Meltzer H (2011) Epidemiology of autism spectrum disorders in adults in the community in England. Arch Gen Psychiatry 68(5):459–465

Brüne M (2005) "Theory of mind" in schizophrenia: a review of the literature. Schizophr Bull 31(1):21–42

Cardno AG, Gottesman II (2000) Twin studies of schizophrenia: from bow-and-arrow concordances to star wars Mx and functional genomics. Am J Med Genet 97(1):12–17

Carroll LS, Owen MJ (2009) Genetic overlap between autism, schizophrenia and bipolar disorder. Genome Med 1(10):102

Cartier E, Hamilton PJ, Belovich AN, Shekar A, Campbell NG et al. 2015. Rareautism-associated variants implicate syntaxin 1 (STX1 R26Q) phosphorylation and the dopamine transporter (hDAT R51W) in dopamine neurotransmission and behaviors. EBioMedicine 2:135–146

Cheung C, Yu K, Fung G, Leung M, Wong C, Li Q, McAlonan G (2010) Autistic disorders and schizophrenia: related or remote? An anatomical likelihood estimation. PLoS One 5(8):e12233

Ching H, Pringsheim T (2012) Aripiprazole for autism spectrum disorders (ASD). Cochrane Database Syst Rev 5

Chung YS, Barch D, Strube M (2014) A meta-analysis of mentalizing impairments in adults with schizophrenia and autism spectrum disorder. Schizophr Bull 40(3):602–616

Ciaramidaro A, Bölte S, Schlitt S, Hainz D, Poustka F, Weber B, Walter H (2015) Schizophrenia and autism as contrasting minds: neural evidence for the hypo-hyper-intentionality hypothesis. Schizophr Bull 41(1):171–179

Cohen IL, Anderson LT, Campbell M (1978) Measurement of drug effects in autistic children. Psychopharmacol Bull 14(4):68–70

Cross-Disorder Group of the Psychiatric Genomics Consortium (2013) Genetic relationship between five psychiatric disorders estimated from genome-wide SNPs. Nat Genet 45(9):984–994

Cooper SA (1997) Psychiatry of elderly compared to younger adults with intellectual disabilities. J Appl Res Intellect Disabil 10(4):303–311

Corcoran C, Davidson L, Sills-Shahar R, Nickou C, Malaspina D, Miller T, McGlashan T (2003) A qualitative research study of the evolution of symptoms in individuals identified as prodromal to psychosis. Psychiatr Q 74(4):313–332

Crespi B, Badcock C (2008) Psychosis and autism as diametrical disorders of the social brain. Behav Brain Sci 31(03):241–261

Daniels JL, Forssen U, Hultman CM, Cnattingius S, Savitz DA, Feychting M, Sparen P (2008) Parental psychiatric disorders associated with autism spectrum disorders in the offspring. Pediatrics 121(5):E1357–E1362. doi:10.1542/peds.2007-2296

Davidson C, Greenwood N, Stansfield A, Wright S (2014) Prevalence of Asperger syndrome among patients of an early intervention in psychosis team. Early Interv Psychiatry 8(2):138–146. doi:10.1111/eip.12039

Davis KL, Stewart DG, Friedman JI, Buchsbaum M, Harvey PD, Hof PR, Haroutunian V (2003) White matter changes in schizophrenia: evidence for myelin-related dysfunction. Arch Gen Psychiatry 60(5):443

Devlin B, Melhem N, Roeder K (2011) Do common variants play a role in risk for autism? Evidence and theoretical musings. Brain Res 1380:78–84

Dickson H, Laurens K, Cullen A, Hodgins S (2011) Meta-analyses of cognitive and motor function in youth aged 16 years and younger who subsequently develop schizophrenia. Psychol Med 1(1):1–13

Dossetor DR (2007) 'All that glitters is not gold': misdiagnosis of psychosis in pervasive developmental disorders – a case series. Clin Child Psychol Psychiatry 12(4):537–548

Eack SM, Bahorik AL, McKnight SA, Hogarty SS, Greenwald DP, Newhill CE, Minshew NJ (2013) Commonalities in social and non-social cognitive impairments in adults with autism spectrum disorder and schizophrenia. Schizophr Res 148(1):24–28

Eaves LC, Ho HH (2008) Young adult outcome of autism spectrum disorders. J Autism Dev Disord 38(4):739–747

Ellison-Wright I, Bullmore E (2009) Meta-analysis of diffusion tensor imaging studies in schizophrenia. Schizophr Res 108(1):3–10

Freitag CM (2006) The genetics of autistic disorders and its clinical relevance: a review of the literature. Mol Psychiatry 12(1):2–22

Goldstein G, Minshew NJ, Allen DN, Seaton BE (2002) High-functioning autism and schizophrenia: a comparison of an early and late onset neurodevelopmental disorder. Arch Clin Neuropsychol 17(5):461–475

Gupta M, Kaur H, Jajodia A, Jain S, Satyamoorthy K, Mukerji M, Kukreti R (2011) Diverse facets of COMT: from a plausible predictive marker to a potential drug target for schizophrenia. Curr Mol Med 11(9):732–743

Hallerback MU, Lugnegard T, Gillberg C (2012) Is autism spectrum disorder common in schizophrenia? Psychiatry Res 198(1):12–17

Hamlyn J, Duhig M, McGrath J, Scott J (2013) Modifiable risk factors for schizophrenia and autism – shared risk factors impacting on brain development. Neurobiol Dis 53:3–9. doi:10.1016/j.nbd.2012.10.023

Hao Y, Liu Z, Jiang T, Gong G, Liu H, Tan L, Zhang Z (2006) White matter integrity of the whole brain is disrupted in first-episode schizophrenia. Neuro Rep 17(1):23–26

Hérault J, Martineau J, Perrot-Beaugerie A, Jouve J, Tournade H, Barthelemy C, Muh J-P (1993) Investigation of whole blood and urine monoamines in autism. Eur Child Adolesc Psychiatry 2(4):211–220

Hofvander B, Delorme R, Chaste P, Nydén A, Wentz E, Ståhlberg O, Gillberg C (2009) Psychiatric and psychosocial problems in adults with normal-intelligence autism spectrum disorders. BMC Psychiatry 9(1):35

Hollis C (2003) Developmental precursors of child-and adolescent-onset schizophrenia and affective psychoses: diagnostic specificity and continuity with symptom dimensions. The Br J Psychiatry 182(1):37–44

Hollis C, Kendall T, Birchwood M et al (2013) Psychosis and schizophrenia in children and young people, vol 155, Clinical Guideline. National Institute for Health and Clinical Excellence, London, pp 1–51

Howes OD, Kapur S (2009) The dopamine hypothesis of schizophrenia: version III – the final common pathway. Schizophr Bull 35(3):549–562

Job DE, Whalley HC, Johnstone EC, Lawrie SM (2005) Grey matter changes over time in high risk subjects developing schizophrenia. Neuroimage 25(4):1023–1030

Joshi G, Petty C, Wozniak J, Henin A, Fried R, Galdo M, Biederman J (2010) The heavy burden of psychiatric comorbidity in youth with autism spectrum disorders: a large comparative study of a psychiatrically referred population. J Autism Dev Disord 40(11):1361–1370

Kaland N, Callesen K, Møller-Nielsen A, Mortensen EL, Smith L (2008) Performance of children and adolescents with Asperger syndrome or high-functioning autism on advanced theory of mind tasks. J Autism Dev Disord 38(6):1112–1123

Kay SR, Flszbein A, Opfer LA (1987) The positive and negative syndrome scale (PANSS) for schizophrenia. Schizophr Bull 13(2):261

Kendler KS, Gallagher TJ, Abelson JM, Kessler RC (1996) Lifetime prevalence, demographic risk factors, and diagnostic validity of nonaffective psychosis as assessed in a US community sample: the national comorbidity survey. Arch Gen Psychiatry 53(11):1022–1031

King BH, Lord C (2011) Is schizophrenia on the autism spectrum? Brain Res 1380:34–41

Kolvin I (1971) Studies in the childhood psychoses: I. Diagnostic criteria and classification. Br J Psychiatry 118(545):381–384

Konstantareas MM, Hewitt T (2001) Autistic disorder and schizophrenia: diagnostic overlaps. J Autism Dev Disord 31(1):19–28

Larsson HJ, Eaton WW, Madsen KM, Vestergaard M, Olesen AV, Agerbo E, Mortensen PB (2005) Risk factors for autism: perinatal factors, parental psychiatric history, and socioeconomic status. Am J Epidemiol 161(10):916–925. doi:10.1093/aje/kwi123

Leekam SR, Nieto C, Libby SJ, Wing L, Gould J (2007) Describing the sensory abnormalities of children and adults with autism. J Autism Dev Disord 37(5):894–910

Lionel AC, Vaags AK, Sato D, Gazzellone MJ, Mitchell EB, Chen HY, Thiruvahindrapuram B (2013) Rare exonic deletions implicate the synaptic organizer Gephyrin (GPHN) in risk for autism, schizophrenia and seizures. Hum Mol Genet 22(10):2055–2066

Lugnegard T, Hallerback MU, Gillberg C (2011) Psychiatric comorbidity in young adults with a clinical diagnosis of Asperger syndrome. Res Dev Disabil 32(5):1910–1917. doi:10.1016/j.ridd.2011.03.025

Marshall M, Rathbone J (2011) Early intervention for psychosis. Schizophr Bull 37(6):1111–1114

McCarthy SE, Makarov V, Kirov G, Addington AM, McClellan J, Yoon S, Krastoshevsky O (2009) Microduplications of 16p11. 2 are associated with schizophrenia. Nat Genet 41(11):1223–1227

McCormick LM, Brumm MC, Beadle JN, Paradiso S, Yamada T, Andreasen N (2012) Mirror neuron function, psychosis, and empathy in schizophrenia. Psychiatry Res Neuroimaging 201(3):233–239

McGlashan TH, Miller TJ, Woods SW (2001) Structured interview for prodromal syndromes (version 3.0). PRIME Research Clinic, Yale School of Medicine, New Haven

Miyamoto S, Miyake N, Jarskog L, Fleischhacker W, Lieberman J (2012) Pharmacological treatment of schizophrenia: a critical review of the pharmacology and clinical effects of current and future therapeutic agents. Mol Psychiatry 17(12):1206–1227

Moreno-De-Luca D, Mulle JG, Kaminsky EB, Sanders SJ, Myers SM, Adam MP, Weik L (2010) Deletion 17q12 is a recurrent copy number variant that confers high risk of autism and schizophrenia. Am J Hum Genet 87(5):618–630

Morgan AJ, Jorm AF (2008) Self-help interventions for depressive disorders and depressive symptoms: a systematic review. Ann Gen Psychiatry 7:13

Morrison A, Hutton P, Wardle M, Spencer H, Barratt S, Brabban A, French P (2012) Cognitive therapy for people with a schizophrenia spectrum diagnosis not taking antipsychotic medication: an exploratory trial. Psychol Med 42(05):1049–1056

Mouridsen S, Rich B, Isager T (2008a) Psychiatric disorders in adults diagnosed as children with atypical autism. A case control study. J Neural Transm 115(1):135–138

Mouridsen SE, Rich B, Isager T (2008b) Epilepsy and other neurological diseases in the parents of children with infantile autism. A case control study. Child Psychiatry Hum Dev 39(1):1–8. doi:10.1007/s10578-007-0062-9

Muck-Seler D, Pivac N, Mustapic M, Crncevic Z, Jakovljevic M, Sagud M (2004) Platelet serotonin and plasma prolactin and cortisol in healthy, depressed and schizophrenic women. Psychiatry Res 127(3):217–226

Mueller S, Keeser D, Reiser M, Teipel S, Meindl T (2012) Functional and structural MR imaging in neuropsychiatric disorders, part 2: application in schizophrenia and autism. Am J Neuroradiol 33(11):2033–2037

Myin-Germeys I, van Os J (2007) Stress-reactivity in psychosis: evidence for an affective pathway to psychosis. Clin Psychol Rev 27(4):409–424

Na Young J, Findling RL (2015) An update on pharmacotherapy for autism spectrum disorder in children and adolescents. Curr Opin Psychiatry 28(2):91–101

Nakamura K, Sekine Y, Ouchi Y, Tsujii M, Yoshikawa E, Futatsubashi M, Suzuki K (2010) Brain serotonin and dopamine transporter bindings in adults with high-functioning autism. Arch Gen Psychiatry 67(1):59–68

Nieminen-von Wendt TS, Metsähonkala L, Kulomäki TA, Aalto S, Autti TH, Vanhala R, von Wendt LO (2004) Increased presynaptic dopamine function in Asperger syndrome. Neuro Rep 15(5):757–760

Nylander L, Gillberg C (2001) Screening for autism spectrum disorders in adult psychiatric out-patients: a preliminary report. Acta Psychiatr Scand 103(6):428–434

Oberman LM, Hubbard EM, McCleery JP, Altschuler EL, Ramachandran VS, Pineda JA (2005) EEG evidence for mirror neuron dysfunction in autism spectrum disorders. Cogn Brain Res 24(2):190–198

Ochoa S, Usall J, Cobo J, Labad X, Kulkarni J (2012) Gender differences in schizophrenia and first-episode psychosis: a comprehensive literature review. Schizophr Res Treat 2012, Article ID 916198

Owen MJ, O'Donovan MC, Thapar A, Craddock N (2011) Neurodevelopmental hypothesis of schizophrenia. Br J Psychiatry 198(3):173–175

Pantelis C, Velakoulis D, McGorry P, Wood S, Suckling J, Phillips L, McGuire P (2003) Neuroanatomical abnormalities before and after onset of psychosis: a cross-sectional and longitudinal MRI comparison. Lancet 361(9354):281

Pilling S, Bebbington P, Kuipers E, Garety P, Geddes J, Orbach G, Morgan C (2002) Psychological treatments in schizophrenia: I. Meta-analysis of family intervention and cognitive behaviour therapy. Psychol Med 32(05):763–782

Puig O, Penadés R, Baeza I, De la Serna E, Sánchez-Gistau V, Bernardo M, Castro-Fornieles J (2014) Cognitive remediation therapy in adolescents with early-onset schizophrenia: a randomized controlled trial. J Am Acad Child Adolesc Psychiatry 53(8):859–868

Rapoport J, Chavez A, Greenstein D, Addington A, Gogtay N (2009) Autism spectrum disorders and childhood-onset schizophrenia: clinical and biological contributions to a relation revisited. J Am Acad Child Adolesc Psychiatry 48(1):10–18

Rossi A, Pollice R, Daneluzzo E, Marinangeli M, Stratta P (2000) Behavioral neurodevelopment abnormalities and schizophrenic disorder: a retrospective evaluation with the Childhood Behavior Checklist (CBCL). Schizophr Res 44(2):121–128

Rutter M (1972) Childhood schizophrenia reconsidered. J Autism Dev Disord 2(3):315–337

Rutter M, Bailey A, Lord C (2003) SCQ: social communication questionnaire. Western Psychological Services, Los Angeles

Sandin S, Lichtenstein P, Kuja-Halkola R, Larsson H, Hultman CM, Reichenberg A (2014) The familial risk of autism. JAMA 311(17):1770–1777

Schneider M, Debbané M, Bassett AS, Chow EW, Fung WLA, van den Bree MB, Kates WR (2014) Psychiatric disorders from childhood to adulthood in 22q11. 2 Deletion Syndrome: results from the international consortium on brain and behavior in 22q11. 2 Deletion Syndrome. Am J Psychiatry 171(6):627–639

Shenton ME, Dickey CC, Frumin M, McCarley RW (2001) A review of MRI findings in schizophrenia. Schizophr Res 49(1):1–52

Smeets F, Lataster T, Hommes J, Lieb R, Wittchen H-U, van Os J (2012) Evidence that onset of psychosis in the population reflects early hallucinatory experiences that through environmental risks and affective dysregulation become complicated by delusions. Schizophr Bull 38(3):531–542

Solomon M, Olsen E, Niendam T, Ragland JD, Yoon J, Minzenberg M, Carter CS (2011) From lumping to splitting and back again: atypical social and language development in individuals with clinical-high-risk for psychosis, first episode schizophrenia, and autism spectrum disorders. Schizophr Res 131(1–3):146–151

Spek AA, Wouters SGM (2010) Autism and schizophrenia in high functioning adults: behavioral differences and overlap. Res Autism Spectr Dis 4(4):709–717. doi:10.1016/j.rasd.2010.01.009

Sporn AL, Addington AM, Gogtay N, Ordoñez AE, Gornick M, Clasen L, Lenane M (2004) Pervasive developmental disorder and childhood-onset schizophrenia: comorbid disorder or a phenotypic variant of a very early onset illness? Biol Psychiatry 55(10):989–994

Sprong M, Becker HE, Schothorst PF, Swaab H, Ziermans TB, Dingemans PM, Van Engeland H (2008) Pathways to psychosis: a comparison of the pervasive developmental disorder subtype Multiple Complex Developmental Disorder and the "At Risk Mental State". Schizophrenia research 99(1):38–47

Stahlberg O, Soderstrom H, Rastam M, Gillberg C (2004) Bipolar disorder, schizophrenia, and other psychotic disorders in adults with childhood onset AD/HD and/or autism spectrum disorders. J Neural Transm 111(7):891–902

Starling J, Dossetor D (2009) Pervasive developmental disorders and psychosis. Curr Psychiatry Rep 11(3):190–196

Stone JM, Morrison PD, Pilowsky LS (2007) Review: glutamate and dopamine dysregulation in schizophrenia – a synthesis and selective review. J Psychopharmacol 21(4):440–452

Sugranyes G, Kyriakopoulos M, Corrigall R, Taylor E, Frangou S (2011) Autism spectrum disorders and schizophrenia: meta-analysis of the neural correlates of social cognition. PLoS One 6(10):e25322

Sullivan PF, Magnusson C, Reichenberg A, Boman M, Dalman C, Davidson M, Långström N (2012) Family history of schizophrenia and bipolar disorder as risk factors for autism family history of psychosis as risk factor for ASD. Arch Gen Psychiatry 69(11):1099–1103

Sullivan S, Rai D, Golding J, Zammit S, Steer C (2013) The association between autism spectrum disorder and psychotic experiences in the Avon longitudinal study of parents and children (ALSPAC) birth cohort. J Am Acad Child Adolesc Psychiatry 52(8):806–814. e802

Tarrier N, Haddock G, Barrowclough C, Wykes T (2002) Are all psychological treatments for psychosis equal? The need for CBT in the treatment of psychosis and not for psychodynamic psychotherapy. Psychol Psychother Theory Res Pract 75(4):365–374

Toal F, Bloemen OJN, Deeley Q, Tunstall N, Daly EM, Page L, Murphy DGM (2009) Psychosis and autism: magnetic resonance imaging study of brain anatomy. Br J Psychiatry 194(5):418–425

van Os J, Hanssen M, Bijl RV, Vollebergh W (2001) Prevalence of psychotic disorder and community level of psychotic symptoms: an urban–rural comparison. Arch Gen Psychiatry 58:663–668

Volkmar FR, Cohen DJ (1991) Comorbid association of autism and schizophrenia. Am J Psychiatry 148(12):1705

Vorstman JAS, Breetvelt EJ, Thode KI, Chow EWC, Bassett AS (2013) Expression of autism spectrum and schizophrenia in patients with a 22q11.2 deletion. Schizophr Res 143(1):55–59. doi:10.1016/j.schres.2012.10.010

Waris P, Lindberg N, Kettunen K, Tani P (2013) The relationship between Asperger's syndrome and schizophrenia in adolescence. Eur Child Adolesc Psychiatry 22(4):217–223

Weiss LA, Shen Y, Korn JM, Arking DE, Miller DT, Fossdal R, Green T (2008) Association between microdeletion and microduplication at 16p11. 2 and autism. N Engl J Med 358(7):667–675

Wing L (1981a) Asperger's syndrome: a clinical account. Psychol Med 11(1):115–129

Wing L (1981b) Sex ratios in early childhood autism and related conditions. Psychiatry Res 5(2):129–37

Wing L (2006) Diagnostic interview for social and communication disorders, 11th edn. Centre for Social and Communication Disorders, Bromley

Winton-Brown TT, Fusar-Poli P, Ungless MA, Howes OD (2014) Dopaminergic basis of salience dysregulation in psychosis. Trends Neurosci 37(2):85–94

Wykes T, Reeder C (2005) Cognitive remediation therapy for schizophrenia. Routledge, London

Yung A, McGorry PD (1996) The prodromal phase of first episode psychosis: past and current phase of first episode psychosis: past and current conceptualisations. Schizophrenia Bulletin Schizophrenia Bulletin 22:353–370

Yung A, Yuen H, McGorry P, Phillips L, Kelly D, Dell'Olio M, Buckby J (2005) Mapping the onset of psychosis: the comprehensive assessment of at-risk mental states. Aust N Z J Psychiatry 39:964–971

Valentina Postorino and Luigi Mazzone

1 Introduction

Feeding and eating disorders (FEDs) are characterized by a markedly abnormal attitude to eating which result in altered pattern of behavior. These include pica, rumination disorder, avoidant/restrictive food intake disorder, anorexia nervosa (AN), bulimia nervosa (BN), and binge-eating disorder (APA 2013). Among FEDs, AN and BN are the most common. AN is an eating disorder diagnosed when an individual body weight is below a minimally normal level (body mass index (BMI) is used for adults, and BMI-for-age percentile is used for children and adolescents) due to a persistent energy intake restriction caused by an intense fear of gaining weight and a disturbance in self-perceived body image (APA 2013). BN is described as recurrent episodes of binge eating generally followed by inappropriate compensatory behaviors in order to prevent weight gain (APA 2013). At first glance, FEDs and autism spectrum disorder (ASD) would appear completely different. However, it is well known that feeding and eating problems, such as atypical eating behaviors at mealtime, are common in individuals with ASD (Cermack et al. 2010; Postorino et al. 2015a). In particular, food selectivity is described as the most frequent one (Cermack et al. 2010; Postorino et al. 2015a). Furthermore, food selectivity is often associated with inadequate nutrient intake, suggesting that a limited diet may put

V. Postorino (✉)
Department of Pediatrics, Marcus Autism Center, Emory University School of Medicine, Atlanta, GA, USA

Department of Neuroscience, I.R.C.C.S. Bambino Gesù Children's Hospital, Child Neuropsychiatry Unit, Rome, Italy
e-mail: valentina.postorino86@gmail.com

L. Mazzone
Department of Neuroscience, I.R.C.C.S. Bambino Gesù Children's Hospital, Child Neuropsychiatry Unit, Rome, Italy
e-mail: gigimazzone@yahoo.it

© Springer International Publishing Switzerland 2016
L. Mazzone, B. Vitiello (eds.), *Psychiatric Symptoms and Comorbidities in Autism Spectrum Disorder*, DOI 10.1007/978-3-319-29695-1_5

any child at risk for nutritional deficiency (Bandini et al. 2010; Bicer and Alsaffar 2013; Schmitt et al. 2008). Literature studies describe that girls with a diagnosis of ASD are at greater risk of developing a FED and males with autism are also at increased risk for low body weight (Kalvya 2009; Oldershaw et al. 2011a, b; Sobanski et al. 1999). Currently, a recent line of research has focused on the hypothesis that there may be an association between FEDs and ASD (Anckarsater et al. 2012; Baron-Cohen et al. 2013; Carton and Smith 2014; Coombs et al. 2011; Courty et al. 2013; Huke et al. 2013, 2014; Mandy and Tchanturia 2015; Rhind et al. 2014; Tchanturia et al. 2013). Specifically, these works have supported the assumption of similar behavioral and cognitive features in FEDs and ASD. For instance, deficits in theory of mind and difficulty in expressing emotions and recognizing emotional stimuli have been reported in individuals with ASD, as well as in patients with AN (APA 2013; Davies et al.,2010; Oldershaw et al. 2010, 2011; Tchanturia et al. 2013). However, given that atypical eating behaviors are common in individuals with ASD, recognizing when these symptoms are reported within the clinical eating disorder range is a challenge for clinicians. Nevertheless, the distinction between these disorders is of crucial importance for the diagnostic and treatment processes. For this reason, practical information for clinicians on the prevalence, phenomenology and clinical features, diagnostic process, neurobiological and genetic bases, and treatment of FEDs in ASD will be described in the present chapter.

2   Prevalence of FEDs in ASD

2.1   Atypical Eating Behaviors and Food Selectivity in ASD

Atypical eating behaviors, and more precisely food selectivity, are often present in children with ASD. Literature studies have shown that this atypical eating behavior is more prevalent in children with ASD than in typically developing children. With these considerations, researches exploring the prevalence of food selectivity in children with ASD have reported highly variable rates, ranging from 13 to 87 % (Ahearn et al. 2001; Bandini et al. 2010; Collins et al. 2003; Cornish 1998; Dominick et al. 2007; Field et al. 2003; Kalvya 2009; Klein and Nowak 1999; Nadon et al. 2011; Schmitt et al. 2008; Schreck and Williams 2006; Schreck et al. 2004; Suarez et al. 2013; Whiteley et al. 2000; Williams et al. 2000, 2005). For instance, Whiteley et al. (2000) reported that 83 % of parents indicated that their children ate a restrictive repertoire of foods as their core diet. Similarly, Williams et al. (2000) found that 67 % of parents reported that their child was a "picky eater." However, 73 % reported that their child had a good appetite for foods that they liked, suggesting that picky eating is not associated with a lack of appetite. On the other hand, Bandini et al. (2010), comparing food selectivity between children with ASD and typically developing children, indicated a lower rate (41.7 %) of this atypical eating behavior in their sample of children with ASD. Of note is that these studies used different definitions of food selectivity; distinct methodologies, including rating scales, checklists, and interviews; as well as daily food record diaries, and this issue may represent a possible explanation for these discrepancies. It's only recent that Bandini et al. (2010) have operationalized the definition of food selectivity to comprise three separate domains: food refusal, limited food repertoire, and high-frequency single food intake (Bandini et al. 2010).

2.2 FEDs in ASD

Studies report highly variable prevalence rates of co-occurring FEDs and ASD ranging from 4 % to 37 % (Anckarsäter et al. 2012; Huke et al. 2013, 2014; Gillberg et al. 1995; Råstam 1992; Råstam et al. 2003; Rhind et al. 2014; Wentz Nilsson et al. 1998, 1999, 2005). It is to note that only two studies evaluated patients with current AN and BN, whereas the remaining were based only on AN samples. Moreover, the majority of studies have investigated retrospectively the presence of an ASD during and following AN (Anckarsäter et al. 2012; Gillberg et al. 1995; Råstam 1992; Råstam et al. 2003; Wentz Nilsson et al. 1998, 2005). For instance, Rastam et al. (2003) evaluating premorbid conditions, including ASD, compared 51 individuals with AN with a group of 51 comparison subjects. These investigators found that 20 % of the sample met the ASD criteria. Moreover, all the researches investigating the comorbidity between these disorders used different screening measures for investigating ASD symptoms; therefore, there is a lack of consistency in terms of methodology that make comparisons between studies difficult.

A recent line of research investigates the presence of autistic traits in AN samples reporting that patients with AN possess high level of autistic-like behaviors (Baron-Cohen et al. 2013; Calderoni et al. 2015; Courty et al. 2013; Hambrook et al 2008; Huke et al. 2013, 2014; Rhind et al. 2014; Tchanturia et al. 2013). For instance, Tchanturia et al. (2013) exploring the association between autistic traits and eating disorder symptoms in a group of 66 participants with AN compared to a group of 66 typical controls found that women with anorexia reported a greater number of autistic traits than typical women. However, it is worth mentioning that all these studies explored the presence of autistic traits in anorexia through a self-report measure (the Autism Spectrum Quotient-AQ); thereby an accurate assessment of autistic traits through gold-standard diagnostic measures for ASD is recommended in future researches (Baron-Cohen et al. 2001).

To our knowledge so far, only one case series investigated the co-occurrence of ASD and AN through the Autism Diagnostic Observation Schedule (ADOS), which is the gold-standard measure for the diagnosis of ASD (Lord et al. 2000; Mandy and Tchanturia 2015). In more detail, Mandy and Tchanturia (2015) evaluating through the ADOS ten women receiving treatment for an eating disorder estimated that seven of them had an ASD. However, it is worth to note that the level of autistic symptoms found in this case series could be overestimated by the fact that one of the participants' inclusion criteria was that an ASD had to be suspected.

3   Phenomenology and Clinical Issues of FEDs in ASD

It is not easy to make a comorbid diagnosis of FED in the context of ASD. In fact, at first glance, these conditions appear to be completely different. FEDs are more common in females than in males, with a female-to-male (F:M) ratio of 10:1 (Smink et al. 2014). Generally, eating disorders begin during adolescence, and the lifetime course and outcomes are highly variable among affected individuals (Anderluh et al. 2009). Indeed, literature studies report that most people with FEDs have an above-average intelligence (Lopez et al. 2010). By contrast, ASD is a lifelong condition with an early onset (12–24 months of age). This condition is more prevalent in males than females, with a M:F ratio of 4:1 (CDC 2014). Moreover, intellectual functioning is one of the factors that contribute to the clinical heterogeneity of this disorder, and literature studies have shown an association between ASD and intellectual disability ranging from 16.4 to 84 % (de Bildt et al. 2004; Miller et al. 2012). Besides these differences, these disorders share some behavioral traits, and several clinical issues make difficult the distinction between these conditions. First, ASD is challenging to identify in females, especially in higher functioning individuals, probably due to a different behavioral phenotype between genders, and it is therefore possible that girls either go undiagnosed or are misdiagnosed (Postorino et al. 2015b). Thus, it could be that behaviors and symptoms used to make a diagnosis are gender specific. A direct consequence of this first diagnostic issue is the fact that the majority of eating disorders can have a later onset compared to autism; thereby, individuals present to adult psychiatrist who may not be able to make the diagnosis. Another issue concerns the fact that starvation itself has a deep impact on brain functioning and can produce a condition that can be misinterpreted as autism, characterized by social retirement, rigidity, and repetitive behaviors (Treasure 2013). Third, children with autism have strong preferences and enjoy repetition (e.g., eating the same foods), as well as sensory sensitivities that may interfere with eating and cause food selectivity. Therefore, distinguishing restricted and repetitive behaviors that are diagnostic features of autism from a more structured eating disorder can be difficult. Indeed, it has to be noticed that when an individual with a FED presents for diagnosis and/or treatment, clinicians often do not investigate the developmental history, which is fundamental in order to make an ASD diagnosis. In fact, generally the first clinical focus is to manage the physical and acute risk of an eating disorder patient. During the diagnostic process, in order to make a clear distinction between these disorders, clinicians have to keep in mind the common behavioral traits of these disorders. For instance, repetitive and rigid behaviors are also present in FEDs and frequently precede the onset of an eating disorder. Obsessive-compulsive features characterized by rigid attitudes and behaviors and problems in set shifting and attention to details have been described in both conditions (Solomon et al. 2008; Tchanturia et al. 2011, 2012). Regarding this last point, it has to be pointed out that in FEDs these features are focused on food and weight, whereas in autism, these are given by repetitive behaviors and narrow interests, which include a range of manifestations according to age and ability (APA 2013). Several studies have described that patients with FEDs have difficulty in recognizing emotional stimuli and expressing emotions, and deficit in theory of mind has been reported in AN and BN samples (Oldershaw et al. 2010, 2011a, b; Davies et al. 2010). As a reminder, although all the features described above are common for both disorders, FEDs are accentuated in the acute illness state and became less pronounced after treatment, whereas in autism these remain stable over time. Social impairments, such as loneliness, shyness, and solitary activities, are often described by clinicians in individuals with a FED, especially in the state that precedes the onset of the disorder (Kim et al. 2009; Krug 2012). It is important to take into account that in order to make a diagnosis of ASD, these impairments in the social abilities must be clearly present since childhood, whereas in case of eating disorders, these are usually circumscribed and time limited and disappear after the management of the acute phase of illness. Thus, a deep assessment of the history and development is necessary in order to distinguish between these disorders and eventually make a comorbid diagnosis.

4 Diagnosis and Evaluation: Assessment Tools

The detection of eating disorders in ASD is particularly challenging for clinicians. Some of the autistic features, such as repetitive behaviors and sensory sensitivity that may interfere with eating, can make the distinction of these disorders even more difficult. Moreover, the diagnostic process is complicated by the fact that adequate tools that might support clinicians in the distinction between these disorders are still lacking. Several studies have investigated food selectivity in autism through different measures (Ahearn et al. 2001; Bandini et al. 2010; Collins et al. 2003; Cornish 1998; Dominick et al. 2007; Field et al. 2003; Kalvya 2009; Klein and Nowak 1999; Nadon et al. 2011; Postorino et al. 2015a; Schmitt et al. 2008; Schreck and Williams 2006; Schreck et al. 2004; Suarez et al. 2013; Whiteley et al. 2000; Williams et al. 2000, 2005). The majority of these studies have used food diaries, parental interviews, nutritional adequacy, and parental standard questionnaires. One of the most commonly used dietary assessment tools is the Food Frequency Questionnaire (FFQ) (Field et al. 1999). It is a self-administered questionnaire that asks participants to report the frequency of consumption and portion size of a series of foods over a defined period of time (e.g., the last month; the last 3 months). However, all these instruments were not specifically created to investigate food selectivity in autistic individuals, thus are probably not appropriate to evaluate these problematic behaviors in ASD. In line with this issue, the measures that are often used to evaluate FEDs are self and parent-report questionnaires not designed for this clinical population. It is important to note that in order to fill these questionnaires, the skills to understand own feelings and problems must be unimpaired. For instance, the most widely self-report questionnaire used to detect FEDs is the Eating Disorder Inventory-3 (EDI-3) (Garner 2004; Giannini et al. 2008). It provides a standardized clinical evaluation of symptomatology associated with eating disorders and consists of 91 items organized into three subscales measuring eating disorder symptoms and nine more general psychological trait subscales. However, even in the presence of average language and cognitive skills, many items of this questionnaire require intact metacognitive abilities. In the same way, parent-report questionnaires or interviews (e.g., the Kiddie–Schedule for Affective Disorders and Schizophrenia–Present and Lifetime version- K-SADS-PL) require the parent to have the ability to discern between the repetitive behaviors typical of autism that may interfere with eating and more structured problems concerning feeding and eating (Kaufman et al. 1997). During the diagnostic process, clinicians have to be aware that since one feature of individuals with ASD is the need to perform ritualistic behaviors, repetitive actions, and routine and structured activities, changes in these routine actions or the discrepancy between social context expectations and autistic functioning can cause in these individuals, especially in high-functioning subjects, stress that may be involved in the development of eating disorders. Therefore, it is possible that FEDs are a consequence of stressful life events (e.g., bereavement, pressure at school, or lack of occupation) in autistic patients showing a predisposition to develop these symptoms. Furthermore, an exacerbation of certain autistic behavioral features related to feeding and eating (i.e., a worsening of food selectivity), as well as changes in the type and pattern of preexisting symptoms, or the onset of new symptoms, in a patient affected by ASD, should warn clinicians and lead them to conduct a more in-depth assessment. In these cases, a complete diagnostic evaluation of FEDs in individuals with ASD should include psychological, physical, and medication management investigations. An initial assessment, in order to collect information on case history, current clinical picture, skills, disabilities, and motor competencies, is important for the diagnostic process of children and adolescents with ASD who develop feeding problems. A broad psychological evaluation on the possible exposure to traumatic or stressful life events should be also undertaken. Moreover, given that girls with autism could be undiagnosed and that feeding and eating problems are sometimes the only and easier clinical signs that bring these patients to a psychiatric service, a good clinical practice is to complete the assessment on all the information described above in patients with FEDs who present severe rigidness and social retirement in order to evaluate the presence of an ASD.

5   Neurobiological Bases and Genetic Overlap

Whether these conditions share neural networks and genes is an important area of research in order to shed light on the mechanisms underlying symptoms and delineate different features of these disorders. Several studies have investigated the neural networks in these two conditions, but to our knowledge, none of these studies have compared brain structures in these clinical populations (Treasure 2013; Zucker et al. 2007). The majority of studies on functional imaging in FEDs have investigated the response to food and body images cues (Van den and Treasure 2009). Recently some functional magnetic resonance imaging researches have provided support that patients with AN, similar to individuals with ASD, report altered activation in brain networks underlying theory of mind, cognitive and behavioral flexibility, and central coherence compared to healthy controls (Fonville et al. 2013;

Schulte-Rüther et al. 2012; Zastrow et al. 2009). Other studies have investigated the biological overlap between these disorders. In particular, some reports have shown a disturbed processing of oxytocin in both AN and ASD (Rastam 1992; Rastam et al. 2003; Tchanturia et al. 2004). Moreover, AN and ASD appear to co-exist within families indicating that these observed similarities may reflect a direct genetic link (Comings and Comings 1991; Gillberg 1985; Steffenburg 1991). However, further studies are needed in order to identify genes that can contribute to the development of these conditions.

6 Treatment

The presence of a comorbid eating disorder in individuals with ASD has direct implication for clinical work. Given that studies describe that patients with FEDs report more autistic traits, shedding light on the social cognitive processing of these patients might be useful in order to predict outcomes and to develop adequate interventions (Baldock and Tchanturia 2007). In fact, difficulties in social functioning may decrease the efficacy of psychological interventions and affect the course of the illness (Treasure et al. 2005). Therefore, a modified psychological therapy for ASD processing styles may improve treatment effectiveness in patients with ASD and a comorbid FED. In the same way, these interventions could be also beneficial for patients with eating disorders and high traits of autism. Programs focusing on promoting social skills in autism have been implemented and have been applied to eating disorders patients. These interventions are based on cognitive behavioral strategies, and even if there is a paucity of randomized control trials (RCT), studies published so far have shown the effectiveness of these psychological therapies in this clinical population (Lock et al. 2013; Galsworthy-Francis and Allan 2014; Tchanturia et al. 2014, 2015). A novel intervention who has shown a growing evidence in the treatment of AN is the cognitive remediation therapy (CRT) (Lock et al. 2013; Tchanturia et al. 2014, 2015). This is a brief manualized intervention (ten sessions) which targets cognitive processes, such as increasing the cognitive flexibility and the ability to switch between mental tasks (set shifting). The literature on this intervention in AN samples consists of single case studies, case series, and four RCTs, which report improvements in all target symptoms and low dropout rates (around 10–15 %) (Brockmeyer et al. 2014; Courty et al 2005; Davies and Tchanturia 2005; Dingemans et al. 2014; Lock et al. 2013; Tchanturia et al. 2007, 2008, 2014). For instance, Dingemans et al. (2014)randomly assigned 82 patients with AN to CRT and treatment as usual or to treatment as usual only. Results showed that patients who received CRT reported a significant improvement in eating disorder symptoms, in quality of life as well as set shifting and central coherence abilities (Dingemans et al. 2014). Although all these studies concur on the efficacy of this intervention in patients with AN, to our knowledge, none of these has investigated the feasibility of the CRT on patients with ASD and co-occurring FEDs. Therefore, further RCTs are needed in order to examine the efficacy of CRT on this clinical population.

Another important topic for the treatment concerns the intervention programs for children with ASD and atypical eating behaviors. Overall, previous studies have demonstrated that trials on behavioral interventions represent a well-supported treatment for children with ASD and food selectivity (Marı'-Bauset et al. 2014; Sharp et al. 2011). In particular, these interventions have shown significant improvements in terms of calorie intake, weight gain, and the variety and volume of food consumed during meals in children with ASD. Recently, a pilot study has investigated the feasibility of a behaviorally based parent training intervention called the "Autism MEAL Plan" to address feeding problems in children with ASD, providing support regarding the utility of the program (Sharp et al. 2014). Given these results, as a good clinical practice, the behavior at meal times should be monitored as part of routine assessments of children with ASD in order to implement the right intervention.

Finally, studies on drug therapy in patients with ASD and a comorbid FED are lacking. Moreover, evidence for drug therapy alone in FEDs is weak (Hay and Claudino 2012). Some trials have reported that low dose of antipsychotic medication can improve symptoms. However, all the studies concur that the intervention for FED patients needs to target both physical (i.e., promotion of weight gain, reducing risk of physical complications) and psychological aspects of the disorder (e.g., working with disordered cognitions, harmful behaviors, body image issues, and associated emotional disturbances) (Galsworthy-Francis and Allan 2014). Therefore, cautions are warranted in the use of pharmacological interventions, and clinicians should explore this possibility only when all the other treatments were worthless.

7　Discussion and Future Directions

Recent studies have highlighted that FEDs can occur in the context of an ASD and that patients with eating disorders report higher degree of autistic traits when compared to healthy controls. However, further researches examining the presence of ASD in FED patients through an in-depth assessment performed by a multidisciplinary team and using gold-standard diagnostic measures for autism (e.g., ADOS) are needed in order to shed light on the prevalence of this comorbidity. Given that in clinical practice the characteristics of the female autistic phenotype are difficult to be recognized, future studies have to address the need of developing proper screening tools for eating disorders specifically designed for the ASD population. Furthermore, whether these two conditions share common cerebral mechanism or genes is still an open issue. In the same way, controlled studies on the medical and psychological treatments of eating disorders in ASD are still lacking. Therefore, we think that it will be important to analyze whether individuals with ASD and FEDs have a distinct etiology, treatment needs, and prognosis compared to people with ASD who do not have FEDs or people with FEDs who do not have ASD. Longitudinal studies might be essential to fill this gap.

References

Ahearn WH, Castine T, Nault K, Green G (2001) An assessment of food acceptance in children with autism or pervasive developmental disorder-not otherwise specified. J Autism Dev Disord 31:505–511

American Psychiatric Association (2013) Diagnostic and statistical manual of mental disorders, 5th edn. American Psychiatric Association, Washington, DC

Anckarsater B, Hofvander E, Billstedt IC, Gillberg C, Gillberg E, Wentz M, Rastam M (2012) The sociocommunicative deficit subgroup in anorexia nervosa: autism spectrum disorders and neurocognition in a community-based, longitudinal study. Psychol Med 42:1957–1967

Anderluh M, Tchanturia K, Rabe-Hesketh S, Collier D, Treasure J (2009) Lifetime course of eating disorders: design and validity testing of a new strategy to define the eating disorders phenotype. Psychol Med 39:105–114

Baldock E, Tchanturia K (2007) Translating laboratory research into practice: foundations, functions and future of cognitive remediation therapy for anorexia nervosa. Future Med 4(3):285–292

Bandini LG, Anderson SE, Curtin C, Cermak S, Evans EW, Scampini R et al (2010) Food selectivity in children with autism spectrum disorders and typically developing children. J Pediatr 157:259–264

Baron-Cohen S, Wheelwright S, Skinner R, Martin J, Clubley E (2001) The autism spectrum quotient (AQ): evidence from Asperger syndrome/high-functioning autism, males and females, scientists and mathematicians. J Autism Dev Disord 31:5–17

Baron-Cohen S, Jaffa T, Davies S, Auyeung B, Allison C, Wheelwright S (2013) Do girls with anorexia nervosa have elevated autistic traits? Mol Autism 4:24

Bicer AH, Alsaffar AA (2013) Body mass index, dietary intake and feeding problems of Turkish children with autism spectrum disorder (ASD). Res Dev Disabil 34:3978–3987

Brockmeyer T, Ingenerf K, Walther S, Wild B, Hartmann M, Herzog W et al (2014) Training cognitive flexibility in patients with anorexia nervosa: a pilot randomized controlled trial of cognitive remediation therapy. Int J Eat Disord 47:24–31

Calderoni S, Fantozzi P, Balboni G, Pagni V, Franzoni E, Apicella F, Narzisi A, Maestro S, Muratori F (2015) The impact of internalizing symptoms on autistic traits in adolescents with restrictive anorexia nervosa. Neuropsychiatr Dis Treat 11:75–85

Carton AM, Smith AD (2014) Assessing the relationship between eating disorder psychopathology and autistic traits in a non-clinical adult population. Eat Weith Disord 19(3):285–293

Cermack SA, Curtin C, Bandini LG (2010) Food selectivity and sensory sensitivity in children with autism spectrum disorders. J Am Diet Assoc 110(2):238–246

Collins MSR, Kyle R, Smith S, Laverty A, Roberts S, Eaton-Evans J (2003) Coping with the usual family diet. Eating behavior and food choices of children with Down's syndrome, autistic spectrum disorders, or Cri du chat syndrome and comparison groups of siblings. J Learn Disabil 7:137–155

Comings DE, Comings BG (1991) Clinical and genetic relationships between autism-pervasive developmental disorder and tourette syndrome: a study of 19 cases. Am J Med Genet 39:180–191

Coombs MS, Bryant-Waugh R, Skevington SM (2011) An investigation into the relationship between eating disorder psychopathology and autistic symptomatology in a non-clinical sample. Br J Clin Psychol 50:326–338

Cornish E (1998) A balanced approach towards healthy eating in autism. J Hum Nutr Diet 11:501–509

Courty ASM, Lalanne C, Ringuenet D, Vindreau C, Chevallier C, Pouga L, Pinabel F, Philippe A, Adrien J, Davies C, Tchanturia K (2005) Cognitive remediation therapy as an intervention for acute anorexia nervosa: a case report. Eur Eat Disord Rev 13:311–316

Courty ASM, Lalanne C, Ringuenet D, Vindreau C, Chevallier C, Pouga L, Pinabel F, Philippe A, Adrien J, Barry C, Berthoz S (2013) Levels of autistic traits in anorexia nervosa: a comparative psychometric study. BMC Psychiatry 13:222

Davies H, Schmidt U, Stahl D, Tchanturia K (2010) Evoked facial emotional expression and emotional experience in people with anorexia nervosa. Int J Eat Disord 44:531–539

De Bildt A, Systema S, Kraijer D, Minderaa R (2004) Prevalence of pervasive developmental disorders in children and adolescents with mental retardation. J Child Psychol Psychiatry 46:275–286

Developmental Disabilities Monitoring Network Surveillance Year 2010 Principal Investigators; Centers for Disease Control and Prevention (CDC) (2014) Prevalence of autism spectrum disorder among children aged 8 years – autism and developmental disabilities monitoring network, 11 sites, United States, 2010. Morbidity and mortality weekly report. Surveill Summ 63(2):1–21

Dingemans AE, Danner UN, Donker JM, Aardoom JJ, van Meer F, Tobias K et al (2014) The effectiveness of cognitive remediation therapy in patients with a severe or enduring eating disorder: a randomized controlled trial. Psychother Psychosom 83:29–36

Dominick KC, Davis NO, Lainhart J, Tager-Flusberg H, Folstein S (2007) Atypical behaviors in children with autism and children with a history of language impairment. Res Dev Disabil 28:145–162

Field AE, Camargo CA, Taylor CB, Berkey CS, Frazier AL, Gillman MW et al (1999) Overweight, weight concerns, and bulimic behaviors among girls and boys. J Am Acad Child Adolesc Psychiatry 38:754–760

Field D, Garland M, Williams K (2003) Correlates of specific childhood feeding problems. J Pediatr Child Health 39:299–304

Fonville L, Lao-Kaim NP, Giampietro V et al (2013) Evaluation of enhanced attention to local detail in anorexia nervosa using the embedded figure test; an fMRI study. PLoS One 8(5):e63964

Galsworthy-Francis L, Allan S (2014) Cognitive behavioral therapy for anorexia nervosa: a systematic review. Clin Psychol Rev 34:54–72

Garner DM (2004) Eating disorder inventory-3. Professional manual. Psychological Assessment Resources, Lutz

Giannini M, Pannocchia L, Dalle Grave R, Muratori F, Viglione V (2008) Eating disorder inventory-3. Giunti OS, Firenze

Gillberg C (1985) Autism and anorexia nervosa: related conditions? Nord J Psychiatry 39:307–312

Gillberg C, Råstam M, Gillberg C (1995) Anorexia nervosa 6 years after onset: part I. Personality disorders. Compr Psychiatry 36:61–69

Hambrook D, Tchanturia K, Schmidt U, Russell T, Treasure J (2008) Empathy, systemizing, and autistic traits in anorexia nervosa: a pilot study. Br J Clin Psychol 47:335–339

Hay PJ, Claudino AM (2012) Clinical psychopharmacology of eating disorders: a research update. Int J Neuropsychopharmacol 15:209–222

Huke V, Turk J, Saeidi S, Kent A, Morgan JF (2013) Autism spectrum disorders in eating disorder populations: a systematic review. Eur J Eating Disord Rev 21(5):345–351

Huke V, Turk J, Saeidi S, Kent A, Morgan JF (2014) The clinical implications of high levels of Autism spectrum disorder features in Anorexia Nervosa: a pilot study. Eur J Eat Disord Rev 22(2):116–121

Kalvya E (2009) Comparison of eating attitudes between adolescent girls with and without asperger syndrome. Daughters' and mothers' report. J Autism Disord 39:480–486

Kaufman J, Birmaher B, Brent D, Rao U, Flynn C, Moreci P, Williamson D, Ryan N (1997) Schedule for affective disorders and schizophrenia for school-age children-present and lifetime version (K-SADS-PL): initial reliability and validity data. J Am Acad Child Adolesc Psychiatry 36(7):980–988

Kim YR, Heo SY, Kang H, Song KJ, Treasure J (2009) Childhood risk factors in Korean women with anorexia nervosa: two sets of case – control studies with retrospective comparisons. Int J Eat Disord 43:598–595

Klein U, Nowak AJ (1999) Characteristics of patients with autistic disorder (AD) presenting for dental treatment. A survey and chart review. Spec Care Dent Off Publ Am Assoc Hosp Dent Acad Dent 19:200–207

Krug I (2012) Low social interactions in eating disorder patients in childhood and adulthood: a multicentre European case control study. J Health Psychol 18:26–37

Lock J, Agras WS, Fitzpatrick KK, Bryson SW, Jo B, Tchanturia K (2013) Is outpatient cognitive remediation therapy feasible to use in randomized clinical trials for anorexia nervosa? Int J Eat Disord 46(6):567–575

Lopez C, Stahl D, Tchanturia K (2010) Estimated intelligence quotient in anorexia nervosa: a systematic review and meta-analysis of the literature. Ann Gen Psychiatry 9:40

Lord C, Risi S, Lambrecht L, Cook EH Jr, Leventhal BL, DiLavore PC et al (2000) The Autism diagnostic observation schedule—generic: a standard measure of social and communication deficits associated with the spectrum of Autism. J Autism Dev Disord 30:205–223

Mandy W, Tchanturia K (2015) Do women with eating disorders who have social and flexibility difficulties really have autism? Acase series. Mol Autism 6:6

Marı'-Bauset S, Zazpe I, Mari-Sanchis A, Llopis-Gonza'lez A, Morales-Sua'rez-Varela M (2014) Food selectivity in autism spectrum disorders: a systematic review. J Child Neurol 29(11):1554–1561

Miller JS, Bilder D, Farley M, Coon H, Pinborough-Zimmerman J, Jenson W et al (2012) Autism spectrum disorder reclassified: a second look at the 1980s Utah/UCLA autism epidemiologic study. J Autism Dev Disord 43:200–210

Nadon G, Feldman DE, Dunn W, Gisel E (2011) Mealtime problems in children with autism spectrum disorder and their typically developing siblings. A comparison study. Autism Int J Res Pract 15:98–113

Oldershaw A, Hambrook D, Tchanturia K, Treasure J, Schmidt U (2010) Emotional theory of mind and emotional awareness in recovered anorexia nervosa patients. Psychosom Med 72(1):73–79

Oldershaw A, Hambrook D, Stahl D, Tchanturia K, Treasure J, Schmidt U (2011a) The socioemotional processing stream in anorexia nervosa. Neurosci Biobehav Rev 35(3):970–988

Oldershaw A, Treasure J, Hambrook D, Tchanturia K, Schmidt U (2011b) Is anorexia nervosa a version of autism spectrum disorders? Eur J Eat Disord Rev 19:462–474

Postorino V, Sanges V, Giovagnoli G, Fatta LM, De Peppo L, Armando M, Vicari S, Mazzone L (2015a) Clinical differences in children with autism spectrum disorder with and without food selectivity. Appetite 1(92):126–132

Postorino V, Fatta LM, De Peppo L, Giovagnoli G, Armando M, Vicari S, Mazzone L (2015b) Longitudinal comparison between male and female preschool children with autism spectrum disorder. J Autism Dev Disord 45(7):2046–2055

Råstam M (1992) Anorexia nervosa in 51 Swedish adolescents: premorbid problems and comorbidity. J Am Acad Child Adolesc Psychiatry 31:5

Råstam M, Gillberg C, Wentz E (2003) Outcome of teenage onset anorexia nervosa in a Swedishcommunity based sample. Eur Child Adolesc Psychiatry 12:78–90

Rhind C, Bonfioli E, Hibbs R, Goddard E, Macdonald P, Gowers S, Schmidt U, Tchanturia K, Micali N, Treasure J (2014) An examination of autism spectrum traits in adolescents with anorexia nervosa and their parents. Mol Autism 5:56

Schmitt L, Heiss C, Campbell E (2008) A comparison of nutrient intake and eating behaviors of boys with and without autism. Top Clin Nutr 23:23–31

Schreck KA, Williams K (2006) Food preferences and factors influencing food selectivity for children with autism spectrum disorders. Res Dev Disabil 27:353–363

Schreck KA, Williams K, Smith AF (2004) A comparison of eating behaviors between children with and without autism. J Autism Dev Disord 34:433–438

Schulte-Rüther M, Mainz V, Fink GR, Herpertz-Dahlmann B, Konrad K (2012) Theory of mind and the brain in anorexia nervosa: relation to treatment outcome. J Am Acad Child Adolesc Psychiatry 51(8):832–841

Sharp WG, Jaquess DL, Morton JF et al (2011) Pediatric feeding disorders: a quantitative synthesis of treatment outcomes. Clin Child Fam Psychol Rev 13:348–365

Sharp WG, Burrell L, Jaquess DL (2014) The autism MEAL plan: a parent-training curriculum to manage eating aversions and low intake among children with autism. Autism 18(6):712–722

Smink FR, van Hoeken D, Oldehinkel AJ, Hoek HW (2014) Prevalence and severity of DSM-5 eating disorders in a community cohort of adolescents. Int J Eat Disord 47(6):610–619

Sobanski E, Marcus A, Henninghausen K, Hebebrand J, Schmidt MH (1999) Further evidence for a low body weight in male children and adolescents with Asperger's disorder. Eur Child Adolesc Psychiatry 8:312–314

Solomon M, Ozonoff SJ, Cummings N, Carter CS (2008) Cognitive control in autism spectrum disorders. Int J Dev Neurosci 26:239–247

Steffenburg S (1991) Neuropsychiatric assessment of children with autism: a population-based study. Dev Med Child Neurol 33:495–511

Suarez MA, Nelson NW, Curtis AB (2013) Longitudinal follow-up of factors associated with food selectivity in children with autism spectrum. The International Journal of Research and Practice, Autism

Tchanturia K, Morris RG, Anderluh MB, Collier DA, Nikolaou V, Treasure J (2004) Set shifting in anorexia nervosa: an examination before and after weight gain, in full recovery and relationship to childhood and adult OCPD traits. J Psychiatr Res 38:545–552

Tchanturia K, Davies H, Campbell IC (2007) Cognitive remediation therapy for patients with anorexia nervosa: preliminary findings. Ann Gen Psychiatry 6:14

Tchanturia K, Davies H, Lopez C, Schmidt U, Treasure J, Wykes T (2008) Letter to the editor: neuropsychological task performance before and after cognitive remediation in anorexia nervosa: a pilot case-series. Psychol Med 38:1371–1373

Tchanturia K, Harrison A, Davies H, Roberts M, Oldershaw A, Nakazato M, Treasure J (2011) Cognitive flexibility and clinical severity in eating disorders. PLoS ONE 6(6):e20462

Tchanturia K, Davies H, Harrison A, Roberts M, Nakazato M, Schmidt U, Treasure J, Morris R (2012) Poor cognitive flexibility in eating disorders: examining the evidence using the Wisconsin cart sorting task. PLoS ONE 7(1):e28331

Tchanturia K, Weineck F, Fidanboylu E, Kern N, Treasure J, Baron Cohen S (2013) Exploring autistic traits in anorexia: a clinical study. Mol Autism 4:44

Tchanturia K, Lounes N, Holttum S (2014) Cognitive remediation in anorexia nervosa and related conditions: a systematic review. Eur J Eat Disord Rev 22:454–462

Tchanturia K, Doris E, Mountfor V, Fleming C (2015) Cognitive Remediation and Emotion Skills Training (CREST) for anorexia nervosa in individual format: self-reported outcomes. BMC Psychiatry 15:53

Treasure J (2013) Coherence and other autistic spectrum traits and eating disorders: building from mechanism to treatment. The Birgit Olsson lecture. Nord J Psychiatry 67:38–42

Treasure J, Tchanturia K, Schmidt U (2005) Research to examine the how rather than the what of change. Couns Psychother Res 5(3):191–202

Van den EF, Treasure J (2009) Neuroimaging in eating disorders and obesity: implications for research. Child Adolesc Psychiatry Clin Am 18:95–115

Wentz Nilsson E, Gillberg C, Råstam M (1998) Familial factors in anorexia nervosa: a community-based study. Compr Psychiatry 39:392–399

Wentz Nilsson E, Gillberg IC, Gillberg C, Råstam M (1999) Ten-year follow-up of adolescent-onset anorexia nervosa: personality disorders. J Am Acad Child Adolesc Psychiatry 38:1389–1395

Wentz Nisson E, Lacey JH, Waller G, Rastam M, Turk J, Gillberg C (2005) Childhood onset neuropsychiatric disorders in adults eating disorder patients. A pilot study. Eur Child Adolesc Psychiatry 14:431–437

Whiteley P, Rodgers J, Shattock P (2000) Feeding patterns in autism. Autism Int J Res Pract 4:207–211

Williams PG, Dalrymple N, Neal J (2000) Eating habits of children with autism. Pediatr Nurs 26:259–264

Williams K, Gibbons BG, Schreck KA (2005) Comparing selective eaters with and without developmental disabilities. J Dev Phys Disabil 17:299–309

Zastrow A, Kaiser S, Stippich C et al (2009) Neural correlates of impaired cognitive-behavioral flexibility in anorexia nervosa. Am J Psychiatry 166(5):608–616

Zucker NL1, Losh M, Bulik CM, LaBar KS, Piven J, Pelphrey KA (2007) Anorexia nervosa and autism spectrum disorders: guided investigation of social cognitive endophenotypes. Psychol Bull 133(6):976–1006

Attention-Deficit Hyperactivity Disorder and Autism Spectrum Disorder

6

Samuele Cortese

1   Introduction

Attention-deficit/hyperactivity disorder (ADHD) is the most common neurodevelopmental disorder (Polanczyk et al. 2014). According to the Diagnostic and Statistical Manual of Mental Disorders, 5th edition, DSM-5 (American Psychiatric Association 2013), ADHD is characterized by a persistent and impairing pattern of inattention and/or hyperactivity/impulsivity. Hyperkinetic disorder (HKD), defined in the International Classification of Diseases, 10th Edition (WHO 1992), is a narrower diagnostic category, requiring both symptoms of inattention and hyperactivity/impulsivity and including individuals diagnosed with the combined presentation of ADHD as per DSM-5 (American Psychiatric Association 2013). A large body of evidence shows that ADHD is often comorbid with other psychiatric conditions, such as oppositional defiant disorder/conduct disorder, specific learning disorders, mood and anxiety disorders, and sleep disturbances (Biederman and Faraone 2005; Cortese et al. 2013). Over the past years, the relationship between attention-deficit/hyperactivity disorder (ADHD), or ADHD symptoms, and autism spectrum disorder (ASD) has been the focus of increasing interest, both from a clinical and research standpoint (Antshel et al. 2013). Criterion E of the previous version of the DSM (DSM-IV-TR) did not allow the comorbid diagnosis of ADHD in individuals with ASD. The underlying rationale was that, since ASD was considered the most severe disorder within the diagnostic hierarchy, any symptoms of inattention and/or hyperactivity/impulsivity were deemed to be an expression of the primary diagnosis of

S. Cortese
Department of Psychology, Developmental Brain-Behaviour Laboratory,
University of Southampton, Southampton, UK

IRCCS Stella Maris, Scientific Institute of Child Neurology and Psychiatry,
Calambrone, Pisa, Italy

The Child Study Center at NYU Langone Medical Center, New York, NY, USA
e-mail: samuele.cortese@gmail.com

© Springer International Publishing Switzerland 2016
L. Mazzone, B. Vitiello (eds.), *Psychiatric Symptoms and Comorbidities in Autism Spectrum Disorder*, DOI 10.1007/978-3-319-29695-1_6

ASD. However, some individuals with ASD do meet full criteria for ADHD, which contributes to a more severe impairment. Moreover, for a subset of individuals with mild ASD (in particular, the condition previously referred to as Asperger's syndrome), the primary reason for clinical referral is ADHD symptoms rather than impairment due to ASD core symptoms. Therefore, it is possible that DSM-IV-TR ADHD criterion E contributed to the undertreatment of impairing ADHD-like symptoms in individuals with ASD. Acknowledging this issue, the most recent version of the DSM (DSM-5) does allow a dual diagnosis of ADHD and ADD, thus highlighting the importance of addressing inattention, hyperactivity, and/or impulsivity in individuals with ASD.

2 Prevalence

ADHD is a major public health issue (Feldman and Reiff 2014). Its worldwide-pooled prevalence is estimated at about 5 % in school-age children (Polanczyk et al. 2007, 2014). Impairing symptoms of ADHD persist in adulthood in up to 65 % of cases (Faraone et al. 2006), with a pooled prevalence of adulthood ADHD around 2.5 % (Simon et al. 2009).

Currently, there are no available meta-analyses on the prevalence of ADHD in individuals with ASD. Across studies, the prevalence of ADHD symptoms in individuals with a primary clinical diagnosis of ASD has been reported to be between 13 and 50 % in the general population and in community-based studies and between 20 and 85 % in clinical samples (Grzadzinski et al. 2011).

3 Phenomenology and Clinical Issues

The main clinical issue when dealing with the recognition and diagnosis of ADHD arguably pertains to the differential diagnosis. Indeed, the core symptoms of ADHD (i.e., inattention, hyperactivity/impulsivity) are highly specific and can characterize several, if not the majority, developmental psychopathological disorders. While the differential diagnosis between ADHD and disorders such as mood and anxiety disorders has been addressed in a large body of research (suggesting that the early onset and chronicity of ADHD should be differentiated from the episodic manifestation of depression/bipolarity and anxiety), the relationships between ADHD and other disorders (such as attachment disorders) need to be better elucidated. Another issue relates to the dimension of "mood dysregulation" that is found in many, although not all, individuals with ADHD. It is currently debated if this dimension should be considered among the defining criteria for ADHD. To complicate the matter, many disorders that can be considered in differential diagnosis with ADHD are claimed to be present also as comorbidity. Arguably, the current atheoretical and descriptive approach of the DSM does not allow to fully disentangle issues pertaining to comorbidity/differential diagnosis in the light of the etiopathophysiology and developmental psychopathology of the symptoms.

4   Peculiar Features of the Disorder in Comorbidity with ASD

4.1   Diagnosis and Evaluation: Assessment Tools

The history/intake interview focusing on the chief complaints about inattention, impulsivity, distractibility, and hyperactivity at school and at home and specifically addressing the DSM-IV criteria for ADHD is the cornerstone of the diagnostic assessment for ADHD (Pliszka 2007). The clinician should perform a detailed interview with the parent(s) about each of the ADHD symptoms listed in DSM-5. For each symptom, the clinician should determine whether it is present as well as its duration, severity, and frequency. Age at onset of the symptoms (<12 years) should be assessed. The patient must have the required number of symptoms, a chronic course, and onset of symptoms during childhood. After reviewing the ADHD symptoms, the clinician should interview the parent(s) regarding other common psychiatric disorders of childhood. Formal structured and semi-structured interviews, such as the Schedule for Affective Disorders and Schizophrenia for School-Age Children (Kaufman et al. 1997), are available. Questionnaires, such as the Conners Parent (Conners et al. 1998b) and Teacher (Conners et al. 1998a) Rating Scales-Revised (CRS-R), are an important and efficient part of the diagnostic assessment but cannot be used in isolation to make a diagnosis of ADHD.

Teachers, parents, and older children can/should all report on symptoms to assess for agreement/validity of diagnosis, to document that the ADHD symptoms occur in multiple settings, and to take advantage of the special information that each can provide. Multiple informants (parents, teachers, youths, and healthcare professionals) do not necessarily agree on diagnosis. If the teacher cannot provide such a rating scale or the parent declines permission to contact the school, then materials from school, such as work samples or report cards, should be reviewed or inquired about. Care must be taken to determine the best interpretation of the data if disagreements occur.

A thorough medical history is part of the initial evaluation. For example, prematurity and frequent episodes of otitis with hearing loss may be risk factors of ADHD. A complete family history for ADHD and its common comorbidities should be taken. ADHD is a highly heritable disorder, and, although a positive family history does not confirm the diagnosis, it can be supportive. After interviewing the parents, the clinician should interview the child or adolescent. Young children are often unaware of their symptoms of ADHD, and older children and adolescents may be aware of symptoms but will minimize their significance. The interview with the child or adolescent allows the clinician to identify signs or symptoms inconsistent with ADHD or suggestive of other serious comorbid disorders. This is achieved by means of a mental status examination, assessing appearance, sensorium, mood, affect, and thought processes. This step is particularly relevant in case of the comorbidity between ADHD and ASD.

Since several medical problems can be associated with ADHD, as previously discussed, the general medical examination is indispensable to corroborate some of these conditions (Nass 2005). The neurologic examination is part of any complete diagnostic evaluation. In addition to the traditional neurologic examination, a number of standardized office examinations that tap developmental neurologic functions are available. Furthermore, the neurologic examination provides an opportunity to evaluate for commonly comorbid neurologic problems of coordination like dyspraxia and dysgraphia (Nass 2005).

Neuropsychological testing is not a necessary part of the diagnostic assessment of ADHD, unless specific comorbid or associated learning issues need to be evaluated. Results of neuropsychological testing, however, may lend support to the diagnosis and are useful to detect possible neuropsychological subtypes that need a targeted management. Intelligence should be assessed. Higher IQ ADHD children may compensate for their attention difficulties sufficiently to mask executive dysfunction on traditional measures.

If the patient's medical history is unremarkable, laboratory or neurological testing is not indicated. The measurement of thyroid levels and thyroid-stimulating hormone should be considered only if symptoms of hyperthyroidism other than increased activity level are present. Exposure to lead, either prenatally or during development, is associated with a number of neurocognitive impairments, including ADHD. If a patient has been raised in environment where exposure to lead paint or plumbing is probable, then serum lead levels should be considered. Serum lead levels, such as measurement of other metals, should not be part of routine screening.

Neuroimaging or genetic studies are not currently indicated in the daily clinical practice (Pliszka 2007).

5   Neurobiological Bases and Genetic Overlap

Increasing evidence from neuroimaging and genetic studies points both to overlap and specificity across the two disorders. A recent review of the literature of structural brain imaging studies [both anatomical magnetic resonance imaging (aMRI) and diffusion tensor imaging (DTI)] concluded that total brain volume (increased in ASD and decreased in ADHD), volume of amygdala (larger in ASD and normal in ADHD), and fractional anisotropy (FA, a DTI proxy of white matter integrity) in the internal capsule (ASD: unclear, ADHD: reduced FA in DTI) differed between the two disorders. By contrast, overlap was reported in the corpus callosum and cerebellum (lower volume in aMRI and decreased FA in DTI) and superior longitudinal fasciculus (reduced FA) (Dougherty et al. 2015). A meta-analysis of from functional magnetic resonance imaging (fMRI) has shown similarities across the two disorders in abnormal activation of regions in the attentional dorsal, executive functions, visual, somatomotor circuits and the default activation circuit and specific deficits in the reward circuit in ADHD and abnormalities in the circuits social cognition and language processes specific to ASD (Proal et al. 2013).

From a genetic standpoint, literature on possible overlaps/differences is still in its infancy. A twin study using twin-based structural equation modeling suggested a moderate phenotypic correlation between autistic and ADHD symptoms. In a bivariate model, genetic correlation (r(g)) between autistic and ADHD traits was 0.72

(Reiersen et al. 2008). The authors concluded that in young adults, a substantial proportion of the genetic influences on self-reported autistic and ADHD symptoms may be shared between the two disorders. Only a few candidate gene studies, linkage studies, and GWAS studies have focused on this co-occurrence, pointing to some promising pleiotropic genes, loci, and single nucleotide polymorphisms (SNPs). For example, a seminal study suggested that 15q QTL has possible pleiotropic effects for ADHD and ASD (Nijmeijer et al. 2010).

6   Treatment

Available treatments for ADHD include pharmacological and non-pharmacological strategies. Pharmacological treatments are an important element of therapeutic strategies for ADHD and are recommended as the first-choice option in several guidelines/practice parameters (e.g., Pliszka 2007), at least for severe cases or as a treatment strategy for patients who have not responded to non-pharmacological interventions (Taylor et al. 2004).

6.1   Pharmacological Treatment

Medications for ADHD include psychostimulant (e.g., methylphenidate and amphetamines) and non-psychostimulant drugs (e.g., atomoxetine or guanfacine). A large body of evidence from randomized controlled trials (RCTs), summarized in several meta-analyses in children and/or adults, shows that psychostimulants [e.g., methylphenidate (Castells et al. 2011; Koesters et al. 2009; Schachter et al. 2001; Van der Oord et al. 2008) or mixed amphetamine salts (Faraone and Biederman 2002) and other amphetamine derivatives (Castells et al. 2011)] are significantly more effective than placebo to control ADHD symptoms, at least in the short term. Indeed, the effect sizes expressing the efficacy of psychostimulants on ADHD core symptoms found in the meta-analysis by Faraone and Buitelaar (2010) (0.72 for methylphenidate and 0.99 for amphetamines) are among the highest ones considering all available pharmacological treatments in psychiatry. Psychostimulants have been found efficacious also when pooling results from studies at longer term (>12 months) (Maia et al. 2014).

Non-psychostimulant treatments, such as atomoxetine (Cheng et al. 2007; Cunill et al. 2013; Kratochvil et al. 2008; Tanaka et al. 2013), are also significantly more efficacious than placebo, at least in the short term, albeit with smaller effect sizes than psychostimulants in terms of efficacy on ADHD core symptoms in the short term (ES: 0.6) (Schwartz and Correll 2014). A meta-analysis (Hanwella et al. 2011) of randomized controlled trials concluded that, overall, methylphenidate and atomoxetine have similar profiles in terms of all-cause discontinuation and incidence of adverse events. However, a recent naturalistic study (Cortese et al. 2015b) showed a better safety profile for methylphenidate than atomoxetine.

There is meta-analytic evidence that when used for ADHD symptoms in children with comorbid ASD, psychostimulants are somewhat less efficacious and less well tolerated than in children with ADHD without ASD. A meta-analysis of four RCTs of methylphenidate for ADHD symptoms in children with ASD found an ES=0.6 (Reichow et al. 2013). The rates of adverse events, including, in particular social withdrawal and irritability, were higher than those typically reported in preschoolers with ADHD without ASD. As for non-psychostimulants, the most recent systematic review of trials of atomoxetine concluded that although clinical practice suggests potential efficacy of atomoxetine for ADHD symptoms in children with ASD, there are not enough controlled clinical trial to corroborate such statement (Ghanizadeh 2013).

6.2   Non-pharmacological Treatments

While medications for ADHD are efficacious in randomized controlled trials (RCT) in the short/medium term and are indicated as the first-line treatment (at least for severe cases, Taylor et al. 2004), they have a number of potential limitations – each affecting some patients. These include (i) partial or nonresponse (Faraone et al. 2006), (ii) possible adverse effects (Cortese et al. 2013), (iii) uncertainty about long-term costs and benefits (Molina et al. 2009), (iv) poor adherence (Adler and Nierenberg 2010), and (v) negative medication-related attitudes from patients, parents, or clinicians (Kovshoff et al. 2012). Therefore, in the past years, there has been an increasing interest to non-pharmacological treatments for ADHD. The most recent and arguably rigorous synthesis of such literature has been carried out in the past 3 years by the European ADHD Guidelines Group (EAGG) in a series of meta-analyses addressing the efficacy of a different number of non-pharmacological treatments for ADHD, including dietary interventions (restricted elimination diets, artificial food color exclusions, and free fatty acid supplementation), behavioral interventions, cognitive training, and neurofeedback. Overall, this series of meta-analyses showed that while all these interventions are efficacious on ADHD core symptoms when considering ratings from assessors probably not blinded, the efficacy of such interventions (with the possible exception for a small effect for free fatty acid supplementation) drops to nonsignificant when relying on rating from blinded assessors (Cortese et al. 2015a; Daley et al. 2014; Sonuga-Barke et al. 2013). However, non-pharmacological interventions have been found efficacious on conditions associated with ADHD. For instance, behavioral interventions had a significant effect on positive parenting, reduction of negative parenting, and on conduct disorders associated with ADHD, also when considering probably blinded ratings (Daley et al. 2014). In addition, cognitive training significantly improved working memory deficits that are impaired in a subsample of children with ADHD (Cortese et al. 2015a).

6.3   Novel Treatment Strategies

Current available treatment approaches for ADHD are symptomatic rather than being grounded on the pathophysiology of the disorder. The search for pathophysiology-based treatments such as transcranial magnetic stimulation (TMS) is ongoing (Zaman 2015), along with the advance in our knowledge on the pathophysiology of the disorder, although at present these therapeutic approaches cannot be recommended as standard and evidence-based treatments for ADHD.

7   Discussion and Future Directions

There are many important questions that should be addressed in future studies. First, further investigation is needed to better understand the reasons underlying the comorbidity between ADHD and ASD. Indeed, since the DSM is conceived as an atheoretical classification, the notion of comorbidity between two disorders is purely meant to be descriptive in order to facilitate the communication among clinicians but does not provide any clue on the possible explanations for this association. Second, genetic and environmental factors and their interaction, underlying the association between ADHD and ASD, deserve further attention. Third, since currently available assessment tools for ADHD do not include items specifically adapted for children with ASD, future research should focus on the evaluation of more specific tools that take into account how the semiology of ADHD is impacted by the co-occurrence of ASD. Finally, specific and, possibly, pathophysiologically based intervention strategies to manage ADHD symptoms in individuals with ADHD are needed, given that standard pharmacological treatments for ADHD are less effective and less well tolerated in individuals with ASD and non-pharmacological therapies for ADHD have been poorly evaluated in this clinical population.

Appendix. Management of Disruptive Behaviors (Other Than ADHD) in Children and Adolescents with ASD

In a sizable portion of patients with ASD referred to child and adolescent mental health services, the main concerns include not only typical ADHD core symptoms (i.e., hyperactivity, inattention, and impulsivity) but also related disruptive behaviors such as physical aggressiveness, temper outbursts, or irritability, the latter being defined as an abnormal disposition to uncontrolled anger or aggression (Elbe and Lalani 2012). Although the prevalence of such maladaptive behaviors has not systematically been evaluated in children/adolescents with ASD, individual studies show that they are frequent and impairing in this population. For example, a study in a sample of 487 young people with pervasive developmental disorder (PDD) showed that up to 30 % of them presented with symptoms of irritability, including aggression (24.5 %), severe tantrums (30.2 %), and deliberate self-injurious behavior (16 %) (Lecavalier 2006).

Empirical evidence is available for both pharmacological and non-pharmacological strategies aimed to manage such impairing behaviors. Non-pharmacological interventions are grounded on behavioral techniques such as stimulus-based procedures (e.g., altering antecedent events), instruction-based procedures (e.g., instruction of appropriate behaviors), extinction-based procedures (e.g., withholding or minimizing presumed reinforcers), reinforcement-based procedures (e.g., increasing desired behaviors), punishment-based procedures (e.g., reducing behavior by delivering a contingent event), and systems change procedures (e.g., altering structural features of environment) (Horner et al. 2002). Although no formal meta-analyses have been published on the efficacy (and safety) of these behavioral interventions, a comprehensive research synthesis concluded that (1) disruption/tantrum was the most likely behavior targeted by such interventions, with aggression being the second most likely; (2) early use of behavioral interventions results in reductions of problem behaviors by 80–90 %; (3) interventions based on functional assessment are more likely to reduce the severity and frequency of disruptive behaviors (Horner et al. 2002).

Another promising and relatively novel intervention is based on Social Stories, originally developed to teach children with autistic spectrum disorders how to play games while increasing their ability to interact with others in a socially appropriate way (Gray 1993). Such stories are written to reflect a situation that the child with ASD finds difficult and provide information on what is happening, why, and which are the desirable responses in that specific social situation. A systematic review of case series reported so far concluded that across all seven research articles retrieved, 13 of 15 participants demonstrated a decrease in the frequency of disruptive behavior, with only two participants recording no change in behavior following the Social Story intervention (Rhodes 2014). It is worthy to point out that a rigorous meta-analysis of the efficacy/effectiveness of non-pharmacological interventions for disruptive behaviors in children with ASD, taking into account the level of blinding of raters, for example, a recent meta-analysis on non-pharmacological interventions for ADHD (Sonuga-Barke et al. 2013), is currently lacking in the field.

With regard to pharmacological treatments, although, as pointed out in the main chapter, no medication is currently approved to treat the core symptoms of ASD, there is an extensive practice, and an increasing evidence base, for the use of several agents to reduce the intensity and frequency of disruptive behaviors associated with ASD. Most of the evidence pertains to antipsychotics, in particular risperidone. The body of research on risperidone for disruptive behaviors has been recently meta-analytically reviewed pooling data from 16 open-label studies and 6 placebo-controlled trials (Sharma and Shaw 2012). This meta-analysis concluded that the sample weighted mean effect size for risperidone was 1.13 for open-label studies and 1.21 for placebo-controlled studies, thus indicating, in both cases, high efficacy of risperidone on ASD-related disruptive behavioral, according to the Cohen's classification of effect size (Cohen 1992). In terms of tolerability and safety, the most common adverse events (AEs) reported in trials of risperidone for ASD included excessive weight gain [e.g., in the Research Units on Pediatric Psychopharmacology (RUPP) study (McDougle et al. 2005): 2.7 ± 2.9 kg vs. 0.8 ± 2.2 kg in the control group], increased appetite, fatigue, drowsiness, dizziness, and drooling. Follow-up data indicate that after 6 months of treatment, risperidone leads to a mean weight gain of about 5 kg, which exceeds developmentally expected norms (Martin et al. 2004). Prolactin levels tend to increase significantly: for instance, after 8 weeks, a fourfold increase has been observed, with a slight decrease after 6 months. Of note, prolactin levels were not associated with any adverse events (Anderson et al. 2007).

Another agent that has been increasingly investigated over the past years is aripiprazole. Two published placebo-controlled randomized trials (Owen et al. 2009; Marcus et al. 2009) assessing the effects of this drug for disruptive behaviors in children with ASD reported a statistically significant reduction of disruptive symptoms favoring aripiprazole (dose: 5–15 mg/day). In the first trial (Owen et al. 2009), discontinuation rates due to adverse events (AEs) were 10.6 % for aripiprazole and 5.9 % for placebo. Extrapyramidal symptom-related AE rates were 14.9 % for aripiprazole and 8.0 % for placebo. Mean weight gain was 2.0 kg with aripiprazole and 0.8 kg with placebo at week 8. No serious AEs were reported. In the second study (Marcus et al. 2009), sedation was the most common AE leading to discontinuation. Presyncope (at the dose of 5 mg/day) and aggression (at 10 mg/day) were the two severe AEs reported during the study. At week 8, mean weight change was +0.3 kg on placebo, +1.3 kg on aripiprazole 5 mg/day, +1.3 kg on aripiprazole 10 mg/day, and 1.5 kg on aripiprazole 15 mg/day.

This body of evidence has led the Food and Drug Administration to approve first risperidone   (www.fda.gov/NewsEvents/Newsroom/PressAnnouncements/2006/ ucm108759.htm) and, more recently, aripiprazole (www.online.lexi.com) for the treatment of irritability associated with autism spectrum disorder in children aged 6–17 years, and by contrast, in Europe, the European Medicines Agency has approved risperidone for the short-term treatment of aggressive or disruptive behaviors in children with subaverage intellectual level and disruptive behavior from the age of 5 years (www.medicines.org.uk/emc/medicine/12818/SPC/).

Other agents that have been assessed for the management of ASD-related disruptive behaviors include typical antipsychotic such as haloperidol [e.g., (Cohen et al. 1980)], although their possible side effects, including sedation, acute dystonia, and withdrawal dyskinesias, do not make this class as first-line option. Research on other drugs, such as antiepileptic (lamotrigine and levetiracetam), amantadine, and carnitine, has not shown so far clear beneficial effects of these agents on disruptive behaviors in children with ASD (Kirino 2014).

With regard to the sequencing of treatments (pharmacological and non-pharmacological), the National Institute for Health and Care Excellence (NICE) guidelines recommended using medication for behavioral problems in ASD only if environmental, psychosocial, or other interventions have been insufficient or cannot be delivered because of the severity of the behavior (https://www.nice.org.uk/guidance/qs51). Many experts in the field [e.g., (Dinnissen et al. 2015; Scahill et al. 2009)] concur with the view that pharmacological treatments should be considered only as short-term option when there is a history of behavioral symptoms that occur in multiple settings and that do not respond to behavioral interventions.

References

Adler LD, Nierenberg AA (2010) Review of medication adherence in children and adults with ADHD. Postgrad Med 122:184–191

American Psychiatric Association (2013) Diagnostic and statistical manual of mental disorders, 5th edn, DSM-5. American Psychiatric Publishing, Washington, DC

Anderson GM, Scahill L, McCracken JT, McDougle CJ, Aman MG, Tierney E et al (2007) Effects of short- and long-term risperidone treatment on prolactin levels in children with autism. Biol Psychiatry 61:545–550

Antshel KM, Zhang-James Y, Faraone SV (2013) The comorbidity of ADHD and autism spectrum disorder. Expert Rev Neurother 13:1117–1128

Biederman J, Faraone SV (2005) Attention-deficit hyperactivity disorder. Lancet 366:237–248

Castells X, Ramos-Quiroga JA, Bosch R, Nogueira M, Casas M (2011a) Amphetamines for Attention Deficit Hyperactivity Disorder (ADHD) in adults. Cochrane Database Syst Rev (6):CD007813

Castells X, Ramos-Quiroga JA, Rigau D, Bosch R, Nogueira M, Vidal X et al (2011a) Efficacy of methylphenidate for adults with attention-deficit hyperactivity disorder: a meta-regression analysis. CNS Drugs 25:157–169

Cheng JY, Chen RY, Ko JS, Ng EM (2007) Efficacy and safety of atomoxetine for attention-deficit/ hyperactivity disorder in children and adolescents-meta-analysis and meta-regression analysis. Psychopharmacology (Berl) 194:197–209

Cohen J (1992) A power primer. Psychol Bull 112:155–159

Cohen IL, Campbell M, Posner D, Small AM, Triebel D, Anderson LT (1980) Behavioral effects of haloperidol in young autistic children. An objective analysis using a within-subjects reversal design. J Am Acad Child Psychiatry 19:665–677

Conners CK, Sitarenios G, Parker JD, Epstein JN (1998a) Revision and restandardization of the Conners Teacher Rating Scale (CTRS-R): factor structure, reliability, and criterion validity. J Abnorm Child Psychol 26:279–291

Conners CK, Sitarenios G, Parker JD, Epstein JN (1998b) The revised Conners' Parent Rating Scale (CPRS-R): factor structure, reliability, and criterion validity. J Abnorm Child Psychol 26:257–268

Cortese S, Holtmann M, Banaschewski T, Buitelaar J, Coghill D, Danckaerts M et al (2013) Practitioner review: current best practice in the management of adverse events during treatment with ADHD medications in children and adolescents. J Child Psychol Psychiatry 54:227–246

Cortese S, Ferrin M, Brandeis D, Buitelaar J, Daley D, Dittmann RW et al (2015a) Cognitive training for attention-deficit/hyperactivity disorder: meta-analysis of clinical and neuropsychological outcomes from randomized controlled trials. J Am Acad Child Adolesc Psychiatry 54:164–174

Cortese S, Panei P, Arcieri R, Germinario EA, Capuano A, Margari L et al (2015b) Safety of methylphenidate and atomoxetine in children with Attention-Deficit/Hyperactivity Disorder (ADHD): data from the Italian National ADHD Registry. CNS Drugs 29(10):865–77

Cunill R, Castells X, Tobias A, Capella D (2013) Atomoxetine for attention deficit hyperactivity disorder in the adulthood: a meta-analysis and meta-regression. Pharmacoepidemiol Drug Saf 22:961–969

Daley D, Van der Oord S, Ferrin M, Danckaerts M, Doepfner M, Cortese S et al (2014) Behavioral interventions in attention-deficit/hyperactivity disorder: a meta-analysis of randomized controlled trials across multiple outcome domains. J Am Acad Child Adolesc Psychiatry 53:835–847

Dinnissen M, Dietrich A, van den Hoofdakker BJ, Hoekstra PJ (2015) Clinical and pharmacokinetic evaluation of risperidone for the management of autism spectrum disorder. Expert Opin Drug Metab Toxicol 11:111–124

Dougherty CC, Evans DW, Myers SM, Moore GJ, Michael AM (2015) A comparison of structural brain imaging findings in autism spectrum disorder and Attention-Deficit Hyperactivity Disorder. Neuropsychol Rev 26(1):25–43

Elbe D, Lalani Z (2012) Review of the pharmacotherapy of irritability of autism. J Can Acad Child Adolesc Psychiatry 21:130–146

Faraone SV, Biederman J (2002) Efficacy of Adderall for attention-deficit/hyperactivity disorder: a meta-analysis. J Atten Disord 6:69–75

Faraone SV, Buitelaar J (2010) Comparing the efficacy of stimulants for ADHD in children and adolescents using meta-analysis. Eur Child Adolesc Psychiatry 19:353–364

Faraone SV, Biederman J, Mick E (2006a) The age-dependent decline of attention deficit hyperactivity disorder: a meta-analysis of follow-up studies. Psychol Med 36:159–165

Faraone SV, Biederman J, Spencer TJ, Aleardi M (2006b) Comparing the efficacy of medications for ADHD using meta-analysis. Med Gen Med 8:4

Feldman HM, Reiff MI (2014) Clinical practice. Attention deficit-hyperactivity disorder in children and adolescents. N Engl J Med 370:838–846

Ghanizadeh A (2013) Atomoxetine for treating ADHD symptoms in autism: a systematic review. J Atten Disord 17:635–640

Gray CA (1993) The original social stories book. Future Horizons, Arlington

Grzadzinski R, Di MA, Brady E, Mairena MA, O'Neale M, Petkova E et al (2011) Examining autistic traits in children with ADHD: does the autism spectrum extend to ADHD? J Autism Dev Disord 41:1178–1191

Hanwella R, Senanayake M, de Silva V (2011) Comparative efficacy and acceptability of methylphenidate and atomoxetine in treatment of attention deficit hyperactivity disorder in children and adolescents: a meta-analysis. BMC Psychiatry 11:176

Horner RH, Carr EG, Strain PS, Todd AW, Reed HK (2002) Problem behavior interventions for young children with autism: a research synthesis. J Autism Dev Disord 32:423–446

Kaufman J, Birmaher B, Brent D, Rao U, Flynn C, Moreci P et al (1997) Schedule for affective disorders and schizophrenia for school-age children-present and lifetime version (K-SADS-PL): initial reliability and validity data. J Am Acad Child Adolesc Psychiatry 36:980–988

Kirino E (2014) Efficacy and tolerability of pharmacotherapy options for the treatment of irritability in autistic children. Clin Med Insights Pediatr 8:17–30

Koesters M, Becker T, Kilian R, Fegert JM, Weinmann S (2009) Limits of meta-analysis: methylphenidate in the treatment of adult attention-deficit hyperactivity disorder. J Psychopharmacol 23:733–744

Kovshoff H, Williams S, Vrijens M, Danckaerts M, Thompson M, Yardley L et al (2012) The decisions regarding ADHD management (DRAMa) study: uncertainties and complexities in assessment, diagnosis and treatment, from the clinician's point of view. Eur Child Adolesc Psychiatry 21:87–99

Kratochvil CJ, Milton DR, Vaughan BS, Greenhill LL (2008) Acute atomoxetine treatment of younger and older children with ADHD: a meta-analysis of tolerability and efficacy. Child Adolesc Psychiatry Ment Health 2:25

Lecavalier L (2006) Behavioral and emotional problems in young people with pervasive developmental disorders: relative prevalence, effects of subject characteristics, and empirical classification. J Autism Dev Disord 36:1101–1114

Maia CR, Cortese S, Caye A, Deakin TK, Polanczyk GV, Polanczyk CA et al (2014) Long-Term efficacy of methylphenidate immediate-release for the treatment of childhood ADHD: a systematic review and meta-analysis. J Atten Disord, in press

Marcus RN, Owen R, Kamen L, Manos G, McQuade RD, Carson WH et al (2009) A placebo-controlled, fixed-dose study of aripiprazole in children and adolescents with irritability associated with autistic disorder. J Am Acad Child Adolesc Psychiatry 48:1110–1119

Martin A, Scahill L, Anderson GM, Aman M, Arnold LE, McCracken J et al (2004) Weight and leptin changes among risperidone-treated youths with autism: 6-month prospective data. Am J Psychiatry 161:1125–1127

McDougle CJ, Scahill L, Aman MG, McCracken JT, Tierney E, Davies M et al (2005) Risperidone for the core symptom domains of autism: results from the study by the autism network of the research units on pediatric psychopharmacology. Am J Psychiatry 162:1142–1148

Molina BS, Hinshaw SP, Swanson JM, Arnold LE, Vitiello B, Jensen PS et al (2009) MTA at 8 years: prospective follow-up of children treated for combined-type ADHD in a multisite study. J Am Acad Child Adolesc Psychiatry 48(5):484–500

Nass RD (2005) Evaluation and assessment issues in the diagnosis of attention deficit hyperactivity disorder. Semin Pediatr Neurol 12:200–216

Nijmeijer JS, Arias-Vasquez A, Rommelse NN, Altink ME, Anney RJ, Asherson P et al (2010) Identifying loci for the overlap between attention-deficit/hyperactivity disorder and autism spectrum disorder using a genome-wide QTL linkage approach. J Am Acad Child Adolesc Psychiatry 49:675–685

Owen R, Sikich L, Marcus RN, Corey-Lisle P, Manos G, McQuade RD et al (2009) Aripiprazole in the treatment of irritability in children and adolescents with autistic disorder. Pediatrics 124:1533–1540

Pliszka S (2007) Practice parameter for the assessment and treatment of children and adolescents with attention-deficit/hyperactivity disorder. J Am Acad Child Adolesc Psychiatry 46:894–921

Polanczyk G, de Lima MS, Horta BL, Biederman J, Rohde LA (2007) The worldwide prevalence of ADHD: a systematic review and metaregression analysis. Am J Psychiatry 164:942–948

Polanczyk GV, Willcutt EG, Salum GA, Kieling C, Rohde LA (2014) ADHD prevalence estimates across three decades: an updated systematic review and meta-regression analysis. Int J Epidemiol 43(2):434–42

Proal E, Gonzalez-Olvera J, Blancas AS, Chalita PJ, Castellanos FX (2013) Neurobiology of autism and attention deficit hyperactivity disorder by means of neuroimaging techniques: convergences and divergences. Rev Neurol 57(Suppl 1):S163–S175

Reichow B, Volkmar FR, Bloch MH (2013) Systematic review and meta-analysis of pharmacological treatment of the symptoms of attention-deficit/hyperactivity disorder in children with pervasive developmental disorders. J Autism Dev Disord 43:2435–2441

Reiersen AM, Constantino JN, Grimmer M, Martin NG, Todd RD (2008) Evidence for shared genetic influences on self-reported ADHD and autistic symptoms in young adult Australian twins. Twin Res Hum Genet 11:579–585

Rhodes C (2014) Do Social Stories help to decrease disruptive behaviour in children with autistic spectrum disorders? A review of the published literature. J Intellect Disabil 18:35–50

Scahill L, Aman MG, McDougle CJ, Arnold LE, McCracken JT, Handen B et al (2009) Trial design challenges when combining medication and parent training in children with pervasive developmental disorders. J Autism Dev Disord 39:720–729

Schachter HM, Pham B, King J, Langford S, Moher D (2001) How efficacious and safe is short-acting methylphenidate for the treatment of attention-deficit disorder in children and adolescents? A meta-analysis. CMAJ 165:1475–1488

Schwartz S, Correll CU (2014) Efficacy and safety of atomoxetine in children and adolescents with attention-deficit/hyperactivity disorder: results from a comprehensive meta-analysis and metaregression. J Am Acad Child Adolesc Psychiatry 53:174–187

Sharma A, Shaw SR (2012) Efficacy of risperidone in managing maladaptive behaviors for children with autistic spectrum disorder: a meta-analysis. J Pediatr Health Care 26:291–299

Simon V, Czobor P, Balint S, Meszaros A, Bitter I (2009) Prevalence and correlates of adult attention-deficit hyperactivity disorder: meta-analysis. Br J Psychiatry 194:204–211

Sonuga-Barke EJ, Brandeis D, Cortese S, Daley D, Ferrin M, Holtmann M et al (2013) Nonpharmacological interventions for ADHD: systematic review and meta-analyses of randomized controlled trials of dietary and psychological treatments. Am J Psychiatry 170:275–289

Tanaka Y, Rohde LA, Jin L, Feldman PD, Upadhyaya HP (2013) A meta-analysis of the consistency of atomoxetine treatment effects in pediatric patients with attention-deficit/hyperactivity disorder from 15 clinical trials across four geographic regions. J Child Adolesc Psychopharmacol 23:262–270

Taylor E, Dopfner M, Sergeant J, Asherson P, Banaschewski T, Buitelaar J et al (2004) European clinical guidelines for hyperkinetic disorder – first upgrade. Eur Child Adolesc Psychiatry 13(Suppl 1):I7–I30

Van der Oord S, Prins PJ, Oosterlaan J, Emmelkamp PM (2008) Efficacy of methylphenidate, psychosocial treatments and their combination in school-aged children with ADHD: a meta-analysis. Clin Psychol Rev 28:783–800

WHO (1992) The ICD-10 classification of mental and behavioral disorders: clinical descriptions and diagnostic guidelines 1992; diagnostic criteria for research 1993. Geneva 1992

Zaman R (2015) Transcranial magnetic stimulation (TMS) in Attention Deficit Hyperactivity Disorder (ADHD). Psychiatr Danub 27(Suppl 1):530–532

Tics and Tourette Syndrome in Autism Spectrum Disorder

7

Alessandro Capuano and Giovanni Valeri

1   Introduction

Autism spectrum disorder (ASD) and Tourette syndrome (TS) are neurodevelopmental disorders that typically begin in childhood and are considered chronic conditions in the lifetime. Even if ASD and TS are apparently different disorders, these two conditions share some epidemiological, phenomenological, and pathophysiological features, and several researchers have considered overlap between ASD and TS. There is an increasing interest in the clinical characteristics and biological underpinnings of TS and common co-occurring psychopathology, including ASD.

Although there is no enough evidence to support a unified theory, recent research has focused on both genetic and neuropathological etiologies of TS and ASD.

ASD is are neurodevelopmental disorder characterized by the presence of impaired social interaction and communication, typically accompanied by restricted interests and/or stereotyped behaviors (American Psychiatric Association, DSM-5 2013). A recent epidemiological study estimated the global prevalence of ASD to be between 1 % and 2 % (Elsabbagh et al. 2012). Comorbid psychiatric disorders are present in 70 % of individuals with ASD (Simonoff et al. 2008): attention deficit hyperactivity disorder (ADHD), obsessive compulsive behaviors/disorder (OCB/D), tics and TS, mood disorders, anxiety, oppositional defiant disorder (ODD), conduct disorder (CD), and personality disorders (PDs).

Tourette syndrome (TS) is the primary tic disorder with an estimated prevalence close to 1 % between 5 and 18 years of age (Burd et al. 2009). Core features of TS are motor and phonic tics (DSM-5). In addition to their well-characterized

A. Capuano
Neurology Unit, Department of Neuroscience,
I.R.C.C.S. Bambino Gesù Children's Hospital, Rome, Italy

G. Valeri (✉)
Child Neuropsychiatry Unit, Department of Neuroscience,
I.R.C.C.S. Bambino Gesù Children's Hospital, Rome, Italy
e-mail: giovanni.valeri@opbg.net

© Springer International Publishing Switzerland 2016
L. Mazzone, B. Vitiello (eds.), *Psychiatric Symptoms and Comorbidities in Autism Spectrum Disorder*, DOI 10.1007/978-3-319-29695-1_7

phenomenology, tics display a peculiar variability over time, which is strongly influenced by a variety of contextual factors. A relevant proportion of patients with TS display complex, tic-like, repetitive behaviors that include echophenomena, coprophenomena, and nonobscene socially inappropriate behaviors (NOSIBs).

Comorbid conditions are ADHD, OCB/D, and ASD; coexistent psychopathologies include depression, anxiety, ODD, CD, and PDs.

The complexity of the Tourette spectrum has been confirmed by cluster and factor analytical approaches (Cavanna et al. 2011). It is suggested that TS is not a unitary condition and that one phenotype ("pure TS" [tics only]) occurs in about 10–14 %.

The presence of comorbid ADHD is the main determinant of cognitive dysfunction in TS patients and influences heavily also the risk of developing disruptive behaviors (Müller-Vahl et al. 2010). The burden of behavioral comorbidities is very important in determining significant impairment, poor self-esteem, and a low quality of life.

2   Prevalence

Epidemiologically, more recent studies have highlighted that ASD is overrepresented in TS, occurring in about 4–5 % of TS population (Burd et al. 2009; Freeman et al. 2000).

Burd et al. (2009) examined 7,288 participants from the Tourette Syndrome International Database Consortium and found that TS substantially increased the risk of ASD/pervasive developmental disorders by 13-fold across the reporting sites.

Furthermore, Kadesjo and Gillberg (2000) found that about 5 % of patients with TS also had a diagnosis of Asperger's syndrome, 17 % showed three or more autistic symptoms, and 65 % had deficits relating to the autism spectrum. Thus, TS and ASD are more frequently associated than expected by chance.

Other common epidemiological features are constituted by (1) gender prevalence, in fact males are considerably more likely to be diagnosed with ASD or TS than females, and (2) age of onset, in fact both disorders often manifest during childhood with the median ages of diagnosis of 4.7 and 6.0 years for ASD and TS, respectively (Centers for Disease Control and Prevention (CDC) Developmental Disabilities Monitoring Network Surveillance Year 2010).

Numerous reports have examined the relationship between ASD and TS (Canitano and Vivanti 2007; Kerbeshian and Larry 2003; Burd et al. 2009; Zappella 2002; Rapin 2001; Baron-Cohen et al. 1999) including several population-based studies identifying a significant relationship between TS and ASD above and beyond what would be expected by chance.

However, highly variable rates of comorbidity between tic disorders and ASD have been reported, ranging from 2.9 to 30 %. This range of incidence rates may be attributed to variable clinical samples and/or differences in research methodology. The association between ASD and tic disorders was initially described in single case reports, followed by several case series presenting an elevated concurrence of ASD and TS as well as examples of tic development positively impacting autistic symptoms in several young children (mostly males). Collectively, these early reports spurred a growing interest and discussion in regard to the potential clinical and genetic overlap between the two disorders.

A consistent limitation in studies reporting overlap between ASD and TS has been capturing large cohorts of TS and/or ASD subjects. In 1999, Baron-Cohen and colleagues identified 8.1 % of 37 school-aged children with autism presenting with comorbid TS (Yang et al. 2012). Later, Canitano et al. evaluated a clinical sample of 105 children with ASD, observing 22 % with a tic disorder (11 % with TS and 11 % with chronic motor tics). These findings suggested that the rate of comorbidity was higher than what would have been expected by chance; however, in both reports, the small sample size limited the generalizability of findings. Recently, the Tourette Syndrome International Consortium was initiated to more accurately describe the comorbidity patterns of TS using a large cohort of individuals. Using these data, (Burd et al. 2009) observed that 4.6 % of the 7,288 participants with TS presented with a comorbid pervasive development disorder (PDD), providing significant support that TS increases the risk for PDD/ASD 13-fold. Further, the presence of TS and comorbid PDD/ASD significantly increased the risk of additional comorbid psychopathology (not including PDD/ASD), with nearly 98 % presenting with one or more comorbidity versus 13.2 % in the group with TS only (Burd et al. 2009). These findings suggest that patients with TS and PDD/ASD may present with a more complex diagnostic picture, likely demanding more comprehensive and intensive managed care.

2.1   Familial and Genetic Findings

Several studies have identified a positive family history of TS and/or ASD in individuals presenting with both disorders concurrently (Mandell et al. 2005; Karagiannidis et al. 2012). In a clinical sample of 105 youth with ASD, Canitano et al. observed a positive family history for tic disorders in 59.5 % of youth presenting with ASD and comorbid TS. Burd et al. also identified an association between neuropsychiatric symptoms (including TS and ASD) and a deletion involving exons 4, 5, and 6 of the gene neuroligin 4 (NLGN4) in a family study.

To further delineate potential genetic associations between TS and ASD, Fernandez et al. (2012) examined gene copy number variants (CNVs) in individuals with TS ($n=460$) compared to control subjects ($n=1,131$). While no significant increases in the number of de novo or transmitted rare CNVs were identified in TS subjects compared to controls, gene mapping within rare CNVs in TS subjects showed significant overlap with CNVs previously identified in individuals with ASD. Taken together, these findings reinforce the idea of a common pathogenetic mechanism and shared genetic risk between the two disorders.

3   Phenomenology and Clinical Issues

3.1   Tourette Syndrome

As defined and widely described, TS is characterized by motor and vocal tics, with a waxing and waning course, often accompanied by compulsive behavior (Cohen et al. 2013). From a phenomenological point of view, tics are classified into "hyperkinetic movement disorders" and they are defined as nonvoluntary body movements or vocal sounds that are made repeatedly, rapidly, and suddenly. Tics are stereotyped but no rhythmic movement. The child or adolescent with a tic experiences it as irresistible but can suppress the movement or noise for a period of time. Both kinds of tics, motor and vocal, can be simple or complex. Simple tics involve only a few muscles or sounds that are not yet words. Examples of simple motor tics include nose wrinkling, facial grimaces, eye blinking, jerking the neck, shrugging the shoulders, or tensing the muscles of the abdomen. Simple vocal tics include grunting, clucking, sniffing, chirping, or throat-clearing noises. Simple tics rarely last longer than a few hundred milliseconds. Complex tics involve multiple groups or muscles or complete words or sentences. Examples of complex motor tics include such gestures as jumping, squatting, making motions with the hands, twirling around when walking, touching or smelling an object repeatedly, and holding the body in an unusual position. Complex motor tics last longer than simple motor tics, usually several seconds or longer. Two specific types of complex motor tics that often cause parents concern are copropraxia, in which the tic involves a vulgar or obscene gesture, and echopraxia, in which the tic is a spontaneous imitation of someone else's movements. Similarly, complex vocal tics involve full speech and language, which may range from the spontaneous utterance of individual words or phrases, such as "Stop," or "Oh boy," to speech blocking or meaningless changes in the pitch, volume, or rhythm of the child's voice. Specific types of complex vocal tics include palilalia, which refers to the child's repetition of his or her own words; coprolalia, which refers to the use of obscene words or abusive terms for certain racial or religious groups; and echolalia, in which the child repeats someone else's last word or phrase. Other features of tics are that they typically occur in bouts or episodes alternating with periods of tic-free behavior lasting from several seconds to several hours. They generally diminish in severity when the child is involved in an absorbing activity such as reading or doing homework and increase in frequency and severity when the child is tired, ill, or stressed. Some children have tics during the lighter stages of sleep or wake up during the night with a tic. Severe complex motor tics carry the risk of physical injury, as the child may damage muscles or joints, fracture bones, or fall down during an episode of these tics. Some children harm themselves deliberately by self-cutting or self-hitting, while others hurt themselves unintentionally by touching or handling lighted matches, razor blades, or other dangerous objects. Severe complex vocal tics may interfere with breathing or swallowing.

3.2   ASD

ASD is defined by qualitative impairments in both communication and social interaction and in restricted and repetitive patterns of behavior, interests, and activities (American Psychiatric Association 2013). Commonly ASD patients present "movement disorders" resembling tics but phenomenologically different called stereotypies. As defined by the Taskforce on Childhood Movement Disorders (Sanger et al. 2010), stereotypies are repetitive, simple movements that can be voluntarily suppressed. Examples include repetitive chewing, rocking, twirling, or touching. These movements can occur also in children with intellectual disability (mental retardation) or other developmental disorders such as Rett syndrome as well as in normal children during neurodevelopment.

Stereotyped and repetitive motor mannerisms or complex whole-body movements (e.g., hand or finger flapping or twisting, rocking, swaying, dipping, walking on tiptoe [toe walking]) are another feature of ASD (Ming et al. 2007; Mandell et al. 2005). Children with ASD may line up an exact number of playthings in the same manner in a stereotyped ritual, without apparent awareness of what the toys represent. Other stereotyped behaviors may include echolalia and idiosyncratic phrases.

Motor mannerisms are reported in 37–95 % of individuals with ASD (Filipek et al. 2000). Motor mannerisms often manifest during the preschool years. Stereotyped motor mannerisms appear to be self-stimulating and may also be self-injurious (Teplin 1999).

Self-injurious behaviors are more common among ASD patients with cognitive disability and include headbanging, face or body slapping, self-biting, or self-pinching. The triggers for these behaviors may be predictable (frustration, anxiety, excitement) or seemingly random.

Sensory processing abilities are aberrant in 42–99 % of individuals with ASD (Filipek et al. 2000). Aberrant responses may include overresponsiveness, underresponsiveness, and paradoxical responses to environmental stimuli (Kientz and Dunn 1997). Examples are (1) visual inspection of objects out of the corner of the eyes; (2) preoccupation with edges, spinning objects, or shiny surfaces, lights, or odors; (3) preoccupation with sniffing or licking nonfood objects; (4) resistance to being touched or increased sensitivity to certain kinds of touch; (5) apparent indifference to pain; (6) strong preferences for and/or compulsive touching of certain textures and strong aversions to others; and (7) hypersensitivity to certain frequencies or types of sound (e.g., distant fire engines) with lack of response to sounds close-by or sounds that would startle other children.

4   Peculiar Features of the Disorder in Comorbidity with ASD

4.1   Similarities in Symptomatology

Beyond potential etiological similarities, phenotypic overlap exists between TS and ASD.

First, there is a significant male predominance in both disorders (approximately 60–80 %).

Second, these disorders have many overlapping clinical symptoms, including social deficits, speech abnormalities (e.g., echolalia or palilalia), sensory abnormalities, obsessive-compulsive symptoms, and repetitive motor behaviors.

However, there are also significant differences between the two disorders, for example, speech abnormalities such as coprolalia may present in TS but are not characteristic of ASD symptoms. In TS, disordered movements present as motor and

Table 7.1 Comparison of *motor* and *nonmotor* features of TS and ASD

	TS	ASD
Motor symptoms	Tics	Stereotypies
	Simple and complex motor tics	Simple and complex stereotypies
	Simple and complex vocal tics	Vocalizations, echolalia
Compulsion, repetitive patterns of behavior	Frequently reported (especially in OCD comorbidity)	Core feature
Impaired socialization	Frequently reported	Core feature
Impaired communication	Frequently reported	Core feature
Impaired attention	Associated symptom	Associated symptom
Hyperactivity	Associated symptom	Associated symptom
Obsessive-compulsive behavior	Associated symptom	Frequently reported
Sensory processing issues	Frequently reported	Associated symptom
Sleep disturbance	Frequently reported	Frequently reported

vocal tics (i.e., repetitive, sudden, brief, irregular, involuntary), while ASD patients often present with stereotypies (i.e., repetitive, ritualistic, rhythmical, purposeful). Further, rigidity and resistance to change, common features of ASD, are somewhat distinct from the classic obsessive symptoms that frequently co-occur with TS.

Specific differences between tics and stereotypies can usually be differentiated by a thorough and comprehensive clinical evaluation, providing an accurate differential diagnosis. A summary of overlapped clinical features of ASD and TS is showed in Table 7.1.

5 Diagnosis and Evaluation: Assessment Tools

The American Psychiatric Association (APA) defined three tic disorders in the 5th edition of the Diagnostic and Statistical Manual of Mental Disorders, or DSM-5: (1) provisional tic disorder, (2) persistent (chronic) motor or vocal tic disorder, and (3) Tourette syndrome. The disorders are distinguished from one another according to three criteria: the child's age at onset, the duration of the disorder, and the number and variety of tics. The diagnosis is based on a set of clinical diagnostic criteria. A classification of tics is shown in Table 7.2.

In particular, TS is defined by the following clinical criteria:

- Both multiple motor tics and one or more phonic tics must be present at some time during the illness, although not necessarily concurrently tics must occur many times a day, nearly every day, or intermittently throughout a period of more than 1 year.
- Onset of tics before the age of 18 years.
- Involuntary movements and noises must not be explained by another medical condition or by the physiological effects of substance.

Table 7.2 Classification of tics

Physiologic tics	Primary pathological tics	Secondary pathological tics ("Tourettism")
Mannerisms	Sporadic	Inherited
	Transient motor or phonic tics (<1 year)	Huntington disease
	Chronic motor or phonic tics (>1 year)	Primary dystonia
	Adult-onset (recurrent) tics	Neuroacanthocytosis
	Tourette syndrome	Neurodegeneration with brain iron accumulation
		Tuberous sclerosis
		Wilson disease
		Infections: encephalitis, Creutzfeldt-Jakob disease, Sydenham chorea
		Drugs: stimulants, levodopa, carbamazepine, phenytoin, phenobarbital, antipsychotics (tardive dyscinesia)
		Toxins: carbon monoxide
		Developmental: static encephalopathy, mental retardation syndromes, chromosomal abnormalities
		Other: head trauma, stroke, neurocutaneous syndromes, schizophrenia, neurodegenerative disorders

5.1   An Integrated Approach to Diagnosis and Evaluation of Tourette and Comorbid Conditions

Based on description made previously in this chapter, it is clear that the diagnosis of TS is based on clinical features of the symptoms. Thus, a detailed medical history and a complete psychosocial and family history to detect psychiatric and/or neurological conditions in relatives are often enough to clarify the clinical framework of the disorder. However, a small minority of patients with TS presents a pure tic disorder, while a psychopathology and comorbidity occur in about 80–90 % (Martino et al. 2013).

A series of scales and other instruments have been developed to completely assess TS and comorbid conditions. An algorithm is shown in Fig. 7.1.

6   Neurobiological Bases and Genetic Overlap

6.1   Neuropathological Similarities

Given the growing evidence suggesting an etiological overlap between TS and ASD, this relationship has been investigated by several researchers via psychopathological, neuropsychological, brain imaging, genetic, and clinical studies.

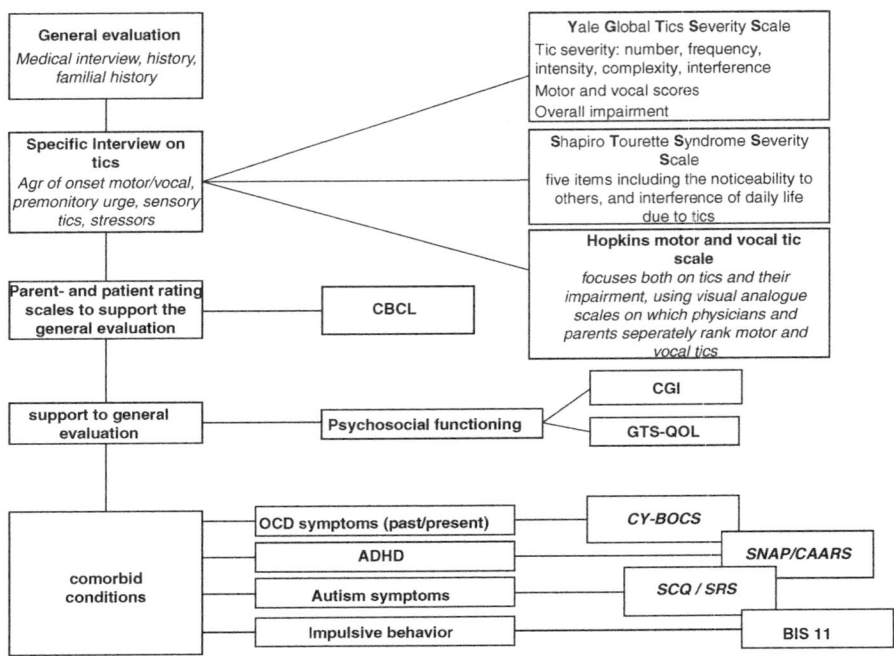

Fig. 7.1 Assessment tool algorithm for TS and its comorbid conditions

A recent review by Kern et al. (2015) observed several neuropsychological similarities between TS, ASD, and ADHD, highlighting that these disorders may be part of a broader neurodevelopmental illness spectrum (termed abnormal connectivity spectrum disorder [ACSD]), resulting from neural processes that cause long-range underconnectivity and short-range overconnectivity. These connectivity abnormalities may be related to neurotoxicity, neuroinflammation, excitotoxicity, sustained microglial activation, proinflammatory cytokines, toxic exposure, and oxidative stress. Evidence also suggests that the severity of connectivity deficits is associated with symptom severity in TS, ASD, and ADHD. Collectively, these data further support the hypothesis that these disorders, though separate, may share common risk factors or possibly etiology.

6.2   Neurobiology of TS and ASD: Common Features and Mechanisms

6.2.1   The Role of Basal Ganglia in TS and ASD

Currently, it is recognized that dysfunctions of basal ganglia (BG) lead to cognitive and behavioral disorders other than purely motor symptoms. Historically, most of reattach attention has been focused on abnormal moments, considering BG as structures purely involved in motor control. It is only since the end of 1990s that cognitive, behavioral, and motivational aspects have been considered as another role of

BG. The implication of BG in behavioral disorders arises from (1) anatomical and functional studies on organization of circuitry into BG, which revealed functional compartmentalization in close relation to different cortical territories; (2) animal models, especially in nonhuman primates that allowed to establish a causal link between dysfunctions in BG and specific motor and nonmotor symptoms; and (3) clinical studies on dopamine therapy or deep brain stimulation (DBS).

As described above, many features of ASD patients represented by gait abnormalities, impairment in dexterity, abnormal/stereotyped movements, and repetitive pattern of behavior suggest an involvement of BG. Moreover, recent experimental and functional studies confirm BG dysfunction in ASD (Shepherd 2013). Thus, BG could be considered the anatomical and functional link between TS and ASD.

6.2.2 BG Anatomy and Recent Theory of Functional Circuitry and Projections

The BG are a complex of deep nuclei that consist of the corpus striatum, globus pallidus (GP), and substantia nigra. The corpus striatum, which includes the caudate nucleus and the putamen, receives input from the cerebral cortex and the thalamus and, in turn, projects to the GP, which projects via the thalamus to the premotor and motor cortex. Thus, in this very simplified view of BG connectivity, we distinguish main input information arising from cortical areas and projected to striatum and a main output pathway arising from GP and directed to cortical areas (primary motor cortex) to facilitate goal-directed movement. Substantia nigra via its dopaminergic pathway modulates GP output. So, one of first model of BG functionality considered different cortical (mainly motor) inputs that converge into only one output pathway controlling the execution of movement (Parent and Hazrati 1995). In 1986, Alexander et al. presented an alternative hypothesis of BG organization with functional parallel loops rather than a unique functional convergence. According to this model, BG are divided into functional territories in close relation to different territories of frontal cortex. The so called cortico-BG circuitry defines a complex pathway in which at least three parallel functional loops can be distinguished: (1) orbitofrontal/anterior cingulate projections to ventral striatum, (2) dorsolateral prefrontal cortex projections to caudate nucleus, and (3) premotor/motor cortex projections to putamen. Projections from BG (output via GPi and substantia nigra) to cortex, mainly through thalamic nuclei constitute a feed-forward circuitry.

Therefore, these three loops process three different domains of movement control. The recognition of relationship between the ventral striatum and the orbitofrontal and cingulate cortices and the return projections to these areas processes the motivational information, the expected outcome and reward (Tremblay et al. 2009). The caudate nucleus and its projection from and to dorsofrontal cortex are related to cognitive aspects regarding the selection of conditioned stimuli that guide action toward the goal (Middleton and Strick 1997). The third loop, the putamen, and motor and premotor cortex related to motor pattern selection and execution. The interaction between these different BG loops could arise from hierarchical corticocortical projections from prefrontal areas to the motor and premotor cortex, providing the link between the three closed parallel loops. In addition, thalamic relay that transmits BG output provides not only a feedback closed-loop but initiates feed-forward open-loop projections to other cortical areas (McFarland and Haber 2002).

On the basis of these anatomical results, these circuits have been divided in several circuits dedicated to more specific cognitive and motor activities, whereas behavioral studies have identified specialized circuits, treating opposite motivational domains according to pleasant or unpleasant stimuli, or processing the motivation for a food reward versus the hedonic value of this reward (Berridge and Kringelbach 2013). The impact of this model is in the view that BG could be implicated in many psychiatric disorders: cognitive aspects of schizophrenia, OCD, ADHD, and phobia and anxiety (Simpson et al. 2010; Yang et al. 2012). TS is a unique model to study BG involvement in motor and nonmotor aspects: a dysfunction of sensory motor territories of BG can be responsible of motor (tics) symptoms, while associative and limbic domains of BG play a role in behavioral (OCD, ADHD) aspects.

Based on the knowledge of BG organization, it has been postulated that in TS patients, a primary dysfunction of striatum leads to an impairment of inhibitory control in BG. Experimental works (Kataoka et al. 2010; Kalanithi et al. 2005) have shown in the brain of TS patients a fewer inhibitory parvalbumin interneurons and cholinergic interneurons in the anterior part of the striatum compared to healthy controls. These interneurons are normally about 1 % of striatal neuronal population but exert a powerful inhibitory control in the striatum. Thus, a hypothesis is that during the neurodevelopment, an impaired migration of these interneurons into the striatum could occur. The final result is a lack of inhibitory control of GP output on cortex. Most of these inhibitory controls inside the striatum allow the selection of relevant information while blocking noise or competitive informations that induce abnormal movement (i.e., tics) or actions inappropriate to context or behaviors.

A systematic review of anatomic imaging studies found that caudate volumes were reduced in children and adults with TS (Plessen et al. 2009). In addition, tic severity in children with TS correlated with sensorimotor cortex volume reduction. Positron emission tomography (PET) scanning has shown variable rates of glucose utilization in basal ganglia as compared with controls. One study, utilizing [18F] fluorodeoxyglucose PET scans, identified a TS-related pattern characterized by increased premotor cortex and cerebellum activity and reduced resting activity of the striatum and orbitofrontal cortex (Pourfar et al. 2011).

6.2.3 The Burden of Genetics in Shared Mechanisms of TS and ASD Pathology

Mainly, five genes have been reported directly disrupted in TS by independent genomic rearrangements and copy number variants with unique breakpoints, namely, IMMPL2, NRNX1, CTNNA3, NLGN4X, and CNTNAP2 (Clarke et al. 2012). Taken into account each isolated gene, it is difficult to interpret genomic disruption related to complex disorders as TS. For example, IMMPL2 is localized into mitochondrial membrane and regulates reactive oxygen levels. However, three of these genes (IMMPL2, NRNX1, and CTNNA3) had undergone recurrent disruption in unrelated TS individuals and other two genes (NLGN4X and CNTNAP2) co-segregate with the disorder within families, which greatly strengthens their pathogenicity. Moreover, the disruption of these genes is associated with comorbid conditions described in TS; in particular, NLGN4X was associated with ASD (Wang et al. 2009). Conversely, all five genes have all shown independent association with ASD (without tics), suggesting their pathogenicity in overlapping phenomenology and epidemiology of TS and ASD.

Polymorphism in two additional structurally related genes LRRN3 and LRRTM3 have shown strong association with ASD susceptibility (Sousa et al. 2010). LRRN3 and LRRTM3 are both neuronal leucine-rich repeat transmembrane protein genes and both interestingly are nested genes. Nested gene is defined as a gene wholly located within another gene, usually in intronic region. LRRN3 and LRRTM3 are nested within two of genes disrupted in TS, i.e., IMMPL2 and CTNNA3, respectively. LRRN3-IMMPL2 and LRRTM3-CTNNA3 may constitute transcriptional complexes in neurodevelopment linking TS and ASD. Both LRR gene-associated proteins are transmembrane proteins involved in synaptic development through protein-protein interactions. They share similar structural domains, particularly the extracellular domain, the LRR domain. LRR domain of LRRTM3 represents a ligand-binding site for the formation of transsynaptic complexes with neurexins (NRXNs). NRXNs are presynaptic proteins that bind neuroligin (NLGNs) and LRRTMs in brain development. NRXN1 gene is disrupted in TS as well as NLGN4X, depicting a complex synaptic interaction in which genetic disruption leads to an imbalance of synaptic formation in TS and ASD (Gauthier et al. 2011). Another gene named CBLN2 has been found associated to TS. CBLN proteins play a role in cell adhesion and synaptogenesis; these proteins bind NRXs and glutamate receptor delta (GRID) competing with NLG-mediated synaptogenesis. Once again, genetic breakdown leads to an imbalance of developmental synaptogenesis (Turrigiano 2012). A summary of genetic findings and their functional implications is reported in Table 7.3.

Table 7.3 Summary of genes involved in TS and ASD and their functional implications

Gene	Locus	Protein encoded	Function
IMMPL2	7q31	Mitochondrial transmembrane protein	Radicals of oxygen regulation
LRRN3 (nested into IMMPL2)	7q31	Leucine-rich repeat neuronal proteins	Postsynaptic protein for protein-protein interaction in synaptogenesis
CTNNA3	10q21	Alpha2-catenin	Transmembrane synaptic ligand
LRRTM3 (nested gene into CTNNA2)	10q21	Leucine-rich repeat transmembrane proteins	Postsynaptic protein neurexins ligand
NRXN1	2p21	Neurexin proteins	Presynaptic transmembrane protein
NRXN4/CNTNAP2	7q35	Neurexin family	Presynaptic transmembrane protein
NLGN4X	Xp22.23	Neuroligin protein family	Postsynaptic neurexin ligand
CBLN2	18q22.2	CBLN superfamily of C1q/tumor necrosis factor superfamily	Neurexin ligand (CBLN2-NRX-GRID complex)

Evidence suggests that neuropathological findings in striatum, the loss of inhibitory interneurons (parvalbumin positive cells) as mentioned above, can be explained by dysfunction of synaptogenesis due to genetic predisposition.

However, phenotypic variability can also be caused by nongenetic factors or second hits such as prematurity, perinatal trauma, hypoxia, infections, autoimmunity, and other modulators such as gender (Herbert 2010).

While the evidence for a genetic contribution is strong, several genes, including SLITRK1, LIM homeobox (LHX6, LHX8), and HDC, have been suggested to be responsible for the different clinical phenotypes (Karagiannidis et al. 2012; Paschou et al. 2012). However, its exact nature has yet to be clarified fully. Etiological factors include genetic vulnerability pre- and perinatal difficulties (PNDs) and probably neuroimmunological factors.

7 Treatment

Treatment of TS and tic disorders includes psychoeducation and reassurance, medications, target-specific botulinum toxin injections, and, in a few severe refractory adult cases, deep brain stimulation life (Müller-Vahl et al. 2011).

General consensus on TS treatment indicates that watch-and-wait strategy works well for many patients with tics. This strategy coupled with psychoeducation improves symptoms tolerance and supports stress reduction. However, a minority of patients needs pharmacological intervention (Roessner et al. 2011). General indications of drug treatment of motor and vocal tics in TS patients include:

1. Subjective discomfort
2. Social isolation or bullying problems
3. Social and emotional problems
4. Functional interference

Thus, the burden of global impairment in daily life is the major indication for medical treatment option. Furthermore, the frequent comorbid conditions associated to TS have to be taken into account for a specific choice of drug.

7.1 Nonmedical Treatments

7.1.1 Behavioral and Psychosocial Intervention

The guidelines from ESSTS Group (Verdellen et al. 2011) were the first European overview describing the state-of-the-art of non-pharmacological evidence-based treatment for tics. The group details two behavioral treatment approaches of different methodology, with most evidence pointing to the effectiveness of habit reversal training (HRT) and exposure with response prevention (ERP), the latter being supported by slightly less evidence in systematic studies. Both interventions are considered first-line behavioral treatments for tics for both children and adults and should be offered to patients. The choice of one or the other therapy will depend on the accessibility of the treatment and the patient's preference.

The rationale behind both therapies is the notion that external and internal physiological factors influence the expression of tics and that tics thus should be regarded as semi-voluntary movements. Along the same lines, tics often are preceded by premonitory urges, and these unpleasant bodily sensations often act as a trigger for tics. Hence, behavioral approaches employ the ability of individuals with TS to actively suppress tics and habituate to the premonitory urges.

HRT comprises a functional analysis of tics and relaxation techniques and psychosocial support activities. This structured and manual-based treatment consists of 6–8 weekly treatment hours over a period of 8–10 weeks. Briefly, the two behavioral approaches follow similar principles, but HRT targets one tic at a time and the method is practiced at specific times of the day, whereas in ERP, the patient is asked to suppress all occurring tics during several times of the day. Although more systematic studies have examined the effectiveness of HRT in clinical settings, effect sizes were larger for ERP than for HRT. In view of the limited benefit of pharmacological treatment and good evidence for the efficacy of HRT, it is worth it to try this form of therapy in children and families who are motivated to start training.

Other treatments that are considered second-line or add-on behavioral treatments mentioned in the review are contingency management, function-based interventions, and relaxation training, whereas neurofeedback in tic disorders is still considered in an experimental stage.

7.2 Pharmacological Interventions

Pharmacotherapy has probably the fastest onset when compared with behavioral treatment options, but few randomized clinical trials exist on pharmacological choices in TS.

The recent guidelines from ESSTS Group (Roessner et al. 2011) reviewed the existing Cochrane reviews and provided the first comprehensive review of medical options through a MEDLINE, Pubmed, and EMBASE search between 1970 and 2010. Based on these guidelines, pharmacological options include antipsychotic agents, noradrenergic agents, and miscellaneous drugs as alternatives. Table 7.4 shows a review of drug classes used in TS and ASD.

Haloperidol, pimozide, and risperidone show the highest level of evidence (receiving a grade A), with several randomized controlled trials (RCTs) showing efficacy for treating tics. First-generation antipsychotics have been associated with adverse effects, including parkinsonism, dystonia, dyskinesia, akathisia, and tardive dyskinesia; thus, the other medications to treat tics are necessary.

Among new (atypical) antipsychotic agents, aripriprazole shows a good profile of tolerability and efficacy. Several nonantipsychotic medications were also recommended for the treatment of tics although most have not been as extensively or as rigorously studied. Among noradrenergic agents, clonidine is used in particular in TS patients with comorbid ADHD. Clonidine resulted efficaciously in reducing tic frequency in randomized controlled trial also in a patch transdermal formulation. Cardiovascular side effects have to be taken into account along with more common side effects as dry mouth, headache, and irritability. Among other drugs used in TS patients, tetrabenazine, a vesicular monoamine transporter type 2 inhibitor, might

Table 7.4 Principal pharmacological treatments for TS and ASD

Drug	TS	ASD	Side effects
Typical neuroleptics			
Haloperidol	Level of evidence A	Useful in reducing mannerisms and stereotypies	EPS, sedation, increased appetite
Pimozide	Level of evidence A	–	EPS, sedation, increased appetite
Atypical neuroleptics			
Aripriprazole	Level of evidence C	Useful in reducing stereotypies	Sedation, akathisia, EPS, headache, increased appetite (lesser than other antipsychotics)
Risperidone	Level of evidence A	Useful in reducing stereotypies	EPS, sedation, increased appetite, orthostatic hypotension
Alpha-adrenergic agonists			
Clonidine	Level of evidence A (ADHD/TS)	–	Sedation, increased appetite, orthostatic hypotension, sleepiness

be an alternative to antipsychotic agents. No tardive dyskinesia or other dystonic side effects have been reported with tetrabenazine.

Recent evidence indicates topiramate as useful alternative for tic reduction, while levetiracetam has not reached enough evidence for its choice in TS treatment. Finally, sertraline should be used in TS/OCD patients.

For the treatment of stereotypies in children with ASD, risperidone has been shown in both a Cochrane review in 2006 and two subsequent randomized control trials to be effective. The addition of pentoxifylline to risperidone may have added benefit.

Haloperidol did not improve stereotypy and was poorly tolerated. There is good evidence that aripiprazole is effective in the treatment of stereotypies in children with ASD.

A large randomized trial of citalopram did not show any improvement in stereotypies. Single trials of levetiracetam, guanfacine, and atomoxetine suggest they are not useful in the reduction of stereotypies in children with ASD.

8   Discussion and Future Directions

Originally described over a century ago, Tourette syndrome is now recognized as a relatively common neurodevelopmental disorder, with a privileged position at the border between neurology and psychiatry. The clinical and epidemiological studies suggest that associated social and emotional/behavioral problems are common in individuals with Tourette syndrome, and it seems likely that the investigation of the neurobiological bases of Tourette syndrome will shed light on the common brain mechanisms underlying movement, social, and behavior regulation.

Overall, ADHD, OCD, depression, personality disorders, and ASD are the most common neuropsychiatric conditions encountered in patients with Tourette syndrome.

Existing research suggests an increased prevalence of comorbid ASD (and/or disturbances in social functioning) among individuals with TS. While the precise nature of these relationships is uncertain, both genetic factors, putative common neurobiological features and co-occurring psychopathology, have been implicated in the etiology and/or maintenance of these difficulties.

Over the last few decades, researchers have identified several factors that may contribute to these social and behavioral disturbances, highlighting the negative impact of comorbid psychiatric diagnoses, disruptive behaviors, and/or increased tic severity. Evidence also suggests that peer victimization experienced by youth with TS is associated with increased tic symptom severity, strength of premonitory urge, loneliness, internalizing symptoms (e.g., anxiety and/or depression), explosive outbursts, and deficits in quality of life.

Although several studies postulate that reducing these disabling social and behavioral aspects of symptom presentations beyond tics will reduce the overall burden of TS, most are cross-sectional or preliminary in nature. As such, interventions for TS, and for TS associated with ASD, should aim to address not only tic severity but also the multifaceted reasons for social and behavioral impairments within this population.

References

Alexander GE, DeLong MR, Strick PL (1986) Parallel organization of functionally segregated circuits linking basal ganglia and cortex. Annu Rev Neurosci 9:357–381

American Psychiatric Association (2013) Diagnostic and statistical manual of mental disorders, fifth edition (DSM-5). American Psychiatric Association, Arlington

Baron-Cohen S, Mortimore C, Moriarty J, Izaguirre J, Robertson M (1999) The prevalence of Gilles de la Tourette's syndrome in children and adolescents with autism. J Child Psychol Psychiatry 40:213–218

Berridge KC, Kringelbach ML (2013) Neuroscience of affect: brain mechanisms of pleasure and displeasure. Curr Opin Neurobiol 23:294–303

Burd L, Li Q, Kerbeshian J, Klug MG, Freeman RD (2009) Tourette syndrome and comorbid pervasive developmental disorders. J Child Neurol 24:170–175

Canitano R, Vivanti G (2007) Tics and Tourette syndrome in autism spectrum disorders. Autism 11:19–28

Cavanna AE, Critchley HD, Orth M, Stern JS, Young MB, Robertson MM (2011) Dissecting the Gilles de la Tourette spectrum: a factor analytic study on 639 patients. J Neurol Neurosurg Psychiatry 82:1320–1323

Clarke RA, Lee S, Eapen V (2012) Pathogenetic model for Tourette syndrome delineates overlap with related neurodevelopmental disorders including Autism. Transl Psychiatry 2:e163

Cohen SC, Leckman JF, Bloch MH (2013) Clinical assessment of Tourette syndrome and tic disorders. Neurosci Biobehav Rev 37:997–1007

Elsabbagh M, Divan G, Koh YJ, Kim YS, Kauchali S, Marcín C, Montiel-Nava C, Patel V, Paula CS, Wang C, Yasamy MT, Fombonne E (2012) Global prevalence of autism and other pervasive developmental disorders. Autism Res 5:160–179

Fernandez TV, Sanders SJ, Yurkiewicz IR, Ercan-Sencicek AG, Kim YS, Fishman DO, Raubeson MJ, Song Y, Yasuno K, Ho WS, Bilguvar K, Glessner J, Chu SH, Leckman JF, King RA,

Gilbert DL, Heiman GA, Tischfield JA, Hoekstra PJ, Devlin B, Hakonarson H, Mane SM, Günel M, State MW (2012) Rare copy number variants in Tourette syndrome disrupt genes in histaminergic pathways and overlap with autism. Biol Psychiatry 1(71):392–402

Filipek PA, Accardo PJ, Ashwal S et al (2000) Practice parameter: screening and diagnosis of autism: report of the Quality Standards Subcommittee of the American Academy of Neurology and the Child Neurology Society. Neurology 55:468–479

Freeman RD, Fast DK, Burd L, Kerbeshian J, Robertson MM, Sandor P (2000) An international perspective on Tourette syndrome: selected findings from 3,500 individuals in 22 countries. Dev Med Child Neurol 2:436–447

Gauthier J, Siddiqui TJ, Huashan P, Yokomaku D, Hamdan FF, Champagne N et al (2011) Truncating mutations in NRXN2 and NRXN1 in autism spectrum disorders and schizophrenia. Hum Genet 130:563–573

Herbert MR (2010) Contributions of the environment and environmentally vulnerable physiology to autism spectrum disorders. Curr Opin Neurol 23:103–110

Kadesjö B, Gillberg C (2000) Tourette's disorder: epidemiology and comorbidity in primary school children. J Am Acad Child Adolesc Psychiatry 39:548–555

Kalanithi PS, Zheng W, Kataoka Y, DiFiglia M, Grantz H, Saper CB, Schwartz ML, Leckman JF, Vaccarino FM (2005) Altered parvalbumin-positive neuron distribution in basal ganglia of individuals with Tourette syndrome. Proc Natl Acad Sci U S A 102:13307–13312

Karagiannidis R, Rizzo Z, Tarnok Z, Wolanczyk T, Hebebrand J, Nöthen MM, Lehmkuhl G, Farkas L, Nagy P, Barta C, Szymanska U, Panteloglou G, Miranda DM, Feng Y, Sandor P, Barr C, TSGeneSEE, Paschou P (2012) Replication of association between a SLITRK1 haplotype and Tourette syndrome in a large sample of families. Mol Psychiatry 17:665–668

Kataoka Y, Kalanithi PS, Grantz H, Schwartz ML, Saper C, Leckman JF, Vaccarino FM (2010) Decreased number of parvalbumin and cholinergic interneurons in the striatum of individuals with Tourette syndrome. J Comp Neurol 518:277–291

Kerbeshian J, Larry B (2003) Tourette syndrome and prognosis in autism. Eur Child Adolesc Psychiatry 12:103

Kern JK, Geier DA, King PG, Sykes LK, Mehta JA, Geier MR (2015) Shared brain connectivity issues, symptoms, and comorbidities in autism spectrum disorder, attention deficit/hyperactivity disorder, and Tourette syndrome. Brain Connect 5:321–335

Kientz MA, Dunn W (1997) A comparison of the performance of children with and without autism on the Sensory Profile. Am J Occup Ther 51:530

Mandell DS, Novak MM, Zubritsky CD (2005) Factors associated with age of diagnosis among children with autism spectrum disorders. Pediatrics 116:1480–1486

Martino D, Madhusudan N, Zis P, Cavanna AE (2013) An introduction to the clinical phenomenology of Tourette syndrome. Int Rev Neurobiol 112:1–33

McFarland NR, Haber SN (2002) Thalamic relay nuclei of the basal ganglia form both reciprocal and nonreciprocal cortical connections, linking multiple frontal cortical areas. J Neurosci 22:8117–8132

Middleton FA, Strick PL (1997) New concepts about the organization of basal ganglia output. Adv Neurol 74:57–68

Ming X, Brimacombe M, Wagner GC (2007) Prevalence of motor impairment in autism spectrum disorders. Brain Dev 29:565–570

Müller-Vahl K, Dodel I, Müller N, Münchau A, Reese JP, Balzer-Geldsetzer M, Dodel R, Oertel WH (2010) Health-related quality of life in patients with Gilles de la Tourette's syndrome. Mov Disord 25:309–314

Müller-Vahl KR, Cath DC, Cavanna AE, Dehning S, Porta M, Robertson MM, Visser-Vandewalle V, ESSTS Guidelines Group (2011) European clinical guidelines for Tourette syndrome and other tic disorders. Part IV: deep brain stimulation. Eur Child Adolesc Psychiatry 20:377

Parent A, Hazrati LN (1995) Functional anatomy of the basal ganglia. I. The cortico-basal ganglia-thalamo-cortical loop. Brain Res Brain Res Rev 20:91–127

Paschou P, Stylianopoulou E, Karagiannidis I, Rizzo R, Tarnok Z, Wolancyzk T, Hebebrand J, Nöthen MM, Lehmkuhl G, Farkas L, Nagy P, Szymanska U, Lykidis D, Androutsos C, Szymanska U, Tsironi V, Koumoula A, Barta C, Klidonas C, Ypsilantis P, Simopoulos P, Skavdis G, Grigoriou M (2012) TSGeneSEE: evaluation of the LIM homeobox genes LHX6 and LHX8 as candidates for Tourette syndrome. Genes Brain Behav 11:444–451

Plessen KJ, Bansal R, Peterson BS (2009) Imaging evidence for anatomical disturbances and neuroplastic compensation in persons with Tourette syndrome. J Psychosom Res 67:559–573

Pourfar M, Feigin A, Tang CC et al (2011) Abnormal metabolic brain networks in Tourette syndrome. Neurology 76:944–952

Rapin I (2001) Autism spectrum disorders: relevance to Tourette syndrome. Adv Neurol 85:89–101

Roessner V, Plessen KJ, Rothenberger A, Ludolph AG, Rizzo R, Skov L, Strand G, Stern JS, Termine C, Hoekstra PJ, ESSTS Guidelines Group (2011) European clinical guidelines for Tourette syndrome and other tic disorders. Part II: pharmacological treatment. Eur Child Adolesc Psychiatry 20:173–196

Sanger TD, Chen D, Fehlings DL, Hallett M, Lang AE, Mink JW, Singer HS, Alter K, Ben Pazi H, Butler EE, Chen R, Collins A, Dayanidhi S, Forssberg H, Fowler E, Gilbert DL, Gorman SL, Gormley ME Jr, Jinnah HA, Kornblau B, Krosschell KJ, Lehman RK, MacKinnon C, Malanga CJ, Mesterman R, Michaels MB, Pearson TS, Rose J, Russman BS, Sternad D, Swoboda KJ, Valero-Cuevas F (2010) Definition and classification of hyperkinetic movements in childhood. Mov Disord 25(11):1538–1549

Shepherd GM (2013) Corticostriatal connectivity and its role in disease. Nat Rev Neurosci 14:278–291

Simonoff E, Pickles A, Charman T, Chandler S, Loucas T, Baird G (2008) Psychiatric disorders in children with autism spectrum disorders: prevalence, comorbidity, and associated factors in a population-derived sample. J Am Acad Child Adolesc Psychiatry 47:921–929

Simpson EH, Kellendonk C, Kandel E (2010) A possible role for the striatum in the pathogenesis of the cognitive symptoms of schizophrenia. Neuron 65:585–596

Sousa I, Clark TG, Holt R, Pagnamenta AT, Mulder EJ, Minderaa RB et al (2010) Polymorphisms in leucine-rich repeat genes are associated with autism spectrum disorder susceptibility in populations of European ancestry. Mol Autism 1:7

Teplin SW (1999) Autism and related disorders. In: Levine MD, Carey WB, Crocker AC (eds) Developmental-behavioral pediatrics, 3rd edn. WB Saunders, Philadelphia

Tremblay L, Worbe Y, Hollerman R (2009) The ventral striatum: a heterogeneous structure involved in reward processing, motivation and decision-making. In: Dr. Dreher JC, Tremblay L (eds) Handbook of reward and decision making. Academic, Oxford, pp 51–77

Turrigiano G (2012) Homeostatic synaptic plasticity: local and global mechanisms for stabilizing neuronal function. Cold Spring Harb Perspect Biol 4:a005736

Verdellen C, van de Griendt J, Hartmann A, Murphy T, ESSTS Guidelines Group (2011) European clinical guidelines for Tourette syndrome and other tic disorders. Part III: behavioural and psychosocial interventions. Eur Child Adolesc Psychiatry 20:197–207

Wang K, Zhang H, Ma D, Bucan M, Glessner JT, Abrahams BS et al (2009) Common genetic variants on 5p14.1 associate with autism spectrum disorders. Nature 459:528–533

Yang H, Spence JS, Devous MD Sr et al (2012) Striatal-limbic activation is associated with intensity of anticipatory anxiety. Psychiatry Res 204:123–131

Zappella M (2002) Early-onset Tourette syndrome with reversible autistic behaviour: a dysmaturational disorder. Eur Child Adolesc Psychiatry 11:18–23

Sleep Disorders and Autism Spectrum Disorder

8

Silvia Miano, Flavia Giannotti, and Flavia Cortesi

1   Introduction

Sleep disorders affect approximately 30 % of typically developing children and decrease to 3–12 % during adolescence (ICSD-3 2014). Sleep disorders may have multidimensional consequences such as poor growth, behavioral and learning problems, and poor quality of family life (ICSD-3 2014). Notwithstanding the significant impact of pediatric sleep disorders, most of them remained worldwide unrecognized, and unresolved. The most common sleep disorders reported by caregivers is chronic insomnia (disorder of initiating and maintaining sleep), behavioral insomnia in most cases, and secondary insomnia due to major sleep problems or other medical issues in the remaining cases (ICSD-3 2014).

The majority of the studies about sleep problems in children with mental disabilities reported unspecific sleep problems such as insomnia, sleep-wake deregulation, or sleepiness. Chronic insomnia (lasting more than 3 months, with sleep onset problems and multiple night awakenings) occurs in about 30–50 % of school-aged children with intellectual disabilities. In addition, epilepsy and other neurological impairments increase the risk and the severity of insomnia and of sleep-wake rhythm disorders (Miano and Peraita-Adrados 2014).

All these considerations are valid also for children with autism spectrum disorder (ASD), considering that in one-quarter of them sleep disorders start from birth (Miano and Ferri 2010). In addition, together with mental delay and epilepsy, sleep disorders are considered early indicators of neurological impairment in ASD (Miano

S. Miano (✉)
Sleep and Epilepsy Center, Neurocenter of Southern Switzerland, Civic Hospital of Lugano, Lugano, Switzerland
e-mail: silvia.miano@gmail.com

F. Giannotti • F. Cortesi
Department of Pediatrics and Developmental Neuropsychiatry,
Center of Pediatric Sleep Disorders, University of Rome La Sapienza, Rome, Italy

© Springer International Publishing Switzerland 2016
L. Mazzone, B. Vitiello (eds.), *Psychiatric Symptoms and Comorbidities in Autism Spectrum Disorder*, DOI 10.1007/978-3-319-29695-1_8

and Ferri 2010). Sleep disorders may exacerbate social interactions, repetitive behaviors, affective problems, and inattention/hyperactivity (Malow et al. 2006a). The relationship between sleep disorders and ASD is complex because circadian abnormalities and epilepsy are strong contributors and have a bidirectional influence on sleep of ASD (Accardo and Malow 2014; Goldman et al. 2014). The importance of these comorbidities with sleep disorders is demonstrated by the significant increasing numbers of papers published during the last two decades, about ASD and sleep. One of the main topic is the role of melatonin in sleep disorders of ASD: It has been reported a disruption and/or reduction of melatonin concentration in urine, plasma, and serum sample both during daytime and nighttime, moreover genes whose products regulate endogenous melatonin and modify sleep patterns have been implicated in the pathogenesis of ASD, and supplemental melatonin has been successfully used to treat sleep onset problems, as evidenced by recent randomized trials in ASD (Veatch et al. 2015; Goldman et al. 2014; Tordjman et al. 2015; Cortesi et al. 2012).

It is desirable in the next future an early management of sleep disorders in ASD, which may influence the prognosis of cognitive and behavioral disabilities. For this reason practical information for clinicians about prevalence, genetic implications, clinical features, diagnostic assessment, and treatment of sleep disorders will be helpful.

2   Prevalence of Sleep Problems in ASD

Sleep problems are particularly common in children with ASD with prevalence rates ranging from 50 % to 80 % compared with a 9–50 % prevalence rates in age-matched typically developing (TD) children (Schreck and Mulick 2000; Wiggs 2001; Polimeni et al. 2005; Doo and Wing 2006; Liu et al. 2006; Malow et al. 2006a, b; Malow and Mc Grew 2008; Richdale and Schreck 2009; Hollway et al. 2011; Kotagal and Broomall 2012). As stated by Ming et al. (2008), they rank as one of the most common concurrent clinical disorders and also one of the most burdensome complaints among parents of children with ASD (Cohen et al. 2014).

It should be noted that some reports revealed an increased proportion of sleep problems in more severely developmentally delayed children (Miano et al. 2007; Giannotti et al. 2008, 2011). However, in a study of highly functioning children with ASD, sleep problems appeared to be relatively specific to them compared with both typically developing and children with intellectual disabilities without autism (Richdale and Prior 1995; Bradley et al. 2004; Couturier et al. 2005). Based on the parental reports, Krakowiak and colleagues (2008) found that 53 % of children (2–5 years in age) with autism had at least one frequently experienced sleep problem compared to 46 % of children with non-ASD developmental delays and 32 % of typically developing children. Moreover, studies comparing children with autism and a history of regression with no developmentally regressed children showed more sleep problems in the regressed than in non-regressed group (Giannotti et al. 2008, 2011).

Sleep disturbances are also persistent in ASD. According to parental reports, up to 63 % of children with ASD and sleep problems reported persistence of their sleep difficulties over a long period of time (Robinson and Richdale 2004). Recently, Hodgle et al. (2014) compared age-related changes in the sleep of children with ASD with those of TD children. Unlike TD children, in which the rate of parental reported sleep disorders dropped significantly with age, in ASD the rate increased from 84 % at 3–5 years to 87 % at 10–17 year of age, with a peak in the middle age group. Interestingly, the type of sleep problems changed with age: while bedtime resistance improved, sleep anxiety worsened significantly with age. Conversely, in May (2015) a 1 year longitudinal study conducted in high-functioning ASD children aged 7–12 years found a slight decrease of sleep disturbances over time (from 78 % to 65 %). Anders et al. (2011) in a longitudinal study on sleep-wake patterns in preschool children with autism, developmental delayed (DD) compared with TD children, reported persistent shorten sleep duration and night-to-night variability in the ASD and DD groups.

Despite variability in definitions of sleep disorders and heterogeneity of ASD patient samples, there is compelling evidence for the high prevalence of sleep disturbances in children with ASD.

3 Phenomenology and Clinical Issues

Children with ASD showed a wide range of sleep problems and many of them experiencing multiple problems concurrently (Delahaye et al. 2014). Interestingly, similar sleep problems occur in all the ASD subgroups, and the only factor associated with a higher risk of sleep problems was the occurrence of them before the age of 2 years (Doo and Wing 2006). The most common sleep problem experienced by children with ASD is insomnia. According to parental reports, sleep onset problems and night wakings commonly occur in children with ASD (Liu et al. 2006; Malow and Mc Grew 2008; Johnson and Malow 2008; Richdale and Schreck 2009; Cortesi et al. 2010). Recently, Engelhartdt et al. (2013) demonstrated that bedroom access to a television or a computer was more strongly associated with reduced sleep in children with ASD compared to TD children. Moreover, compared to TD, ASD children spend more time playing video games and watching TV, having more troubles disengaging from screen-based media (Nally et al. 2000). This increased media use coupled with the potential influence of bright screens on melatonin production and circadian rhythms (Engelhardt et al. 2013). A recent meta-analysis study based on objective measures confirm a prolonged sleep latency, shortened sleep duration, and less sleep efficiency in children with autism, even though these alterations are more common in those with concurrent intellectual disability (Elrod and Hoods 2015). Lengthy periods of nocturnal awakening lasting for up to 2–3 h have been reported when the child may simply laugh, talk, scream, or get up and play with toys or various objects in the room (Robinson and Richdale 2004; Malow et al. 2006b; Miano et al. 2007; Goodlin-Jones et al. 2008; Giannotti et al. 2011). As noted by

Richdale and Schreck 2009, these types and duration of night wakings seem typical for children with autism.

The etiology of insomnia in children with autism is thought to be multifactorial, including potential disruption in circadian rhythms and melatonin dysregulation besides poor sleep hygiene practices (Richdale and Schreck 2009; Johnson and Malow 2008). Particularly, fragmented irregular sleep-wake patterns, including inconsistent sleep onset and rise time, free-running sleep-wake rhythm, sleep onset delay, and early morning awakening have been reported (Wiggs and Stores 2004; Goodlin-Jones et al. 2008; Richdale and Schreck 2009; Giannotti et al. 2011). Furthermore, children with autism showed a marked night-to-night variability in their sleep-wake cycle (Anders et al. 2011). Moreover, Matsuura and colleagues (2008) experimentally reproduced sleep patterns of autistic children and suggested a bifurcation of the sleep-wake cycle with increased sensitivity to external noise and short sleep duration.

A recent study showed that insomnia in children with autism may be due to arousal dysregulation and sensory over-responsivity (Mazurek et al. 2015). An over-responsivity to sensory input within the sleep environment, including noise, light, and temperature, was significantly associated with sleep onset delay, sleep duration, and night waking in these children. As reported by Richdale et al. (2014) in ASD children, pre-sleep cognitive arousal was associated with insomnia by increasing physiological arousal and emotional distress which interfere with sleep. Moreover, Tordjman et al. (2014) found a flattened circadian rhythm of cortisol, suggesting also alterations in circadian time structure in children with autism.

Furthermore, children with ASD may be more prone to insomnia due to the neurobiologic overlap with other concurrent medical and psychiatric problems. Epilepsy, which occurs in a significant minority of patients with ASD, may negatively impact sleep (Giannotti et al. 2008; Accardo and Malow 2014).

4   Peculiar Features of Sleep Disorders in Comorbidity with ASD and Impact of Other Comorbidities to Sleep Problems

Psychiatric comorbidity and epilepsy may worsen the management and prognosis of sleep disorders in ASD. In addition, the differential diagnosis between primary insomnia and sleep major disorders remains a challenging diagnosis for clinicians, especially in children with mental disabilities and ASD. Major sleep disorders (such as restless legs syndrome, nocturnal epilepsy, sleep disordered breathing) should always be suspected in ASD children with insomnia not respondent to standard treatment and who display multiple awakenings during sleep and hypersomnia during daytime (although normal hours of bedtime have been demonstrated).

The aim of this paragraph is not reporting in details the pathogenesis and implications of psychiatric comorbidity of ASD, but clinicians should take in mind that psychiatric disorders may worsen insomnia and that specific sleep problems may anticipate the onset of psychiatric disorders (such as attention-deficit hyperactivity disorders, bipolar disorders, anxiety, depression, and psychosis). A brief summary of sleep problems in these specific psychiatric disorders will be helpful for better management of both disorders (ASD and psychiatric comorbidity). Anxiety and depression are recognized as major co-occurring problems in children and young people with ASD. The state of hypervigilance or hyperarousal, which represents the main sign of anxiety, strongly and negatively influence sleep, as it has been also widely describe in psychophysiological insomnia (Ivanenko and Johnson 2008). Children with anxiety disorders may complain of severe sleep onset and maintenance problems, frequent nocturnal awakenings, bedtime refusal, cosleeping, nightmares, and nocturnal fears. Anxiety is strongly associated with specific sleep habits: sleeping with the lights on, requiring a toy/object for sleep onset, sensitivity to noises, fear of the dark or of being alone, and requiring bedtime rituals (Ivanenko and Johnson 2008). On the contrary, early final awakening is a strong indicator of the onset of a major depressive disorder, especially during prepubertal and pubertal age (Ivanenko and Johnson 2008). Recent studies showed that children with autism and co-occurring anxiety may be particularly predisposed to sleep problems (Nadeau et al. 2014; Mazurek et al. 2015). As stated by Nadeau et al. (2014), anxiety symptoms may impact children's sleep in multiple ways. First, it may significantly impact bedtime routine, especially if anxiety is centered around bedtime with fear of dark and separation. Second, physiological symptoms of anxiety such as heart palpitation, sweating, etc. could contribute to exacerbate sleep insomnia (Nadeau et al. 2014). As hypothesized by Mazurek et al. (2015), children with ASD and anxiety may have trouble falling asleep due to increased physiological arousal and autonomic activity. Sedative antidepressant, such as trazodone, may be warranted in cases of depressive symptoms or anxiety disorder associated with insomnia, resistant to cognitive-behavioral therapy (Owens et al. 2010), and this may be also valid in children with ASD.

About 30 % of ASD patients have comorbid attention-deficit hyperactivity disorders (ADHD), with clinically significant levels of ADHD symptoms, particularly hyperactivity. However, there are also comorbid children with a primary ADHD diagnosis and significant social interaction problems (Chantiluke et al. 2014). This bidirectional interaction between ASD and ADHD is also reflected in the allowance for co-diagnosis in the Association AP (2013). While it is well recognized that ADHD and ASD share common deficits in executive functions (EF) (Rommelse et al. 2011), children with ASD may also share the same sleep phenotype described in children with ADHD (Miano et al. 2013). About 25–50 % of children and adolescents with attention-deficit hyperactivity disorder (ADHD) experience sleep problems. According to literature data, five sleep phenotypes may be identified: a sleep phenotype characterized mainly by a hypo-arousal state, resembling narcolepsy, a phenotype associated with delayed sleep onset latency and with a higher risk of bipolar disorder, a phenotype associated with sleep disordered breathing (SDB), another phenotype related to restless legs syndrome (RLS) and/or periodic limb movements (PLMDs), lastly, a phenotype related to epilepsy/or EEG interictal discharges. These major sleep disorders described in children with ADHD have been poorly reported in children with ASD and/or with intellectual disabilities (Miano et al. 2007, 2013), although sleep fragmentations caused by sleep disorders induce early in life and in some cases irreversible frontal and prefrontal deficits (Miano et al. 2013). It is strongly suggested to explore and exclude the presence of major sleep disorders or of nocturnal epilepsy in children with ASD, especially with comorbid ADHD and referred sleep problems. Although is a very rare condition, some children with narcolepsy and cataplexy, especially after the H1N1 pandemic influenza or vaccination, may have florid psychotic symptoms due to signs and symptoms of cataplexy and to many hypnagogic hallucinations during daytime, inducing both ADHD and ASD symptoms and misleading diagnosis (Rocca et al. 2015).

Furthermore, an association between sleep problems and gastrointestinal dysfunction has been described in children with ASD (Johnson 2005; Ming et al. 2008).

While children with ASD do not appear to be particularly at an increased risk for obstructive sleep apnea, other sleep problems, such as parasomnias, may be likely underdiagnosed. Research regarding the prevalence of parasomnias in the autistic population is mixed with some studies suggesting an increased prevalence and others demonstrating no increase (Richdale and Prior 1995; Patzold et al. 1998; Schreck and Mulick 2000; Liu et al. 2006; Wiggs and Stores 2004). There are mixed reports regarding the association of REM sleep behavior disorder (RBD) with autism too. RBD was reported to occur in a number of children with ASD described in a case series (Thirumalai et al. 2002). Additionally, a relatively high percentage of periodic leg movements during sleep has been reported in children with autism (Dosman et al. 2007).

The report of frequent multiple awakening, sleepiness, nocturnal hyperkinesia, and/or stereotyped and clinic movements during sleep may be suspected of nocturnal seizures. Epilepsy is more common in ASD patients than in the general pediatric population, with the prevalence rates estimated at 2–3 % among all children compared with 30 % in ASD, even in children with ASD without other risks for epilepsy (normal intelligence; no family history; no other risk factors, such as cerebral palsy and perinatal disorders; or other medical disorders) (Malow 2006). In the absence of a history of clinical seizures, interictal epileptiform discharges (IEDs) also are more prevalent in ASD patients (Malow 2006). It has been demonstrated that approximately 32 % of children with epilepsy evaluated using validated autism screening questionnaires fit the criteria for having ASD. Most of these children had not been previously diagnosed and have the worst behavior, early occurrence seizures (approximately 2 years), more difficulty falling back to sleep after arousals, early morning wakings, and daytime sleepiness (Clarke 2005). Therefore children with ASD and epilepsy should particularly be evaluated for sleep disturbances (Accardo and Malow 2014). It has been reported a higher percentage of regression and of sleep problems in ASD children with epilepsy and in those with frequent EEG epileptiform activity compared with those with rare or no abnormalities (Giannotti et al. 2008). The coexistence of disrupted sleep patterns and epilepsy in regressed children suggests a disruption of the neuronal circuitry, since the peak age at onset of sleep problems coincides with that of regression, during the second year of life. In ASD, prolonged EEG recording including sleep showed increased prevalence of IEDs (up to 60 % of cases), especially over temporal regions, only seen during sleep (Chez et al. 2006), or over frontal regions (Valdizán-Usón et al. 2002). Interestingly, magnetoelectroencephalography identified more frequently epileptiform activity (82 % of cases) compared to the EEG recording (68 % of cases) (Lewine et al. 1999). The same intra-/perisylvian epileptiform regions of Landau-Kleffner syndrome were active in the majority of cases but also additional nonsylvian zones of independent epileptiform activity were recorded (Lewine et al. 1999).

5   Diagnosis and Evaluation: Assessment Tools

Sleep problems in children with ASD have been widely investigated by sleep questionnaires, and actigraphic recording (usually associated with sleep diaries), more rarely with polysomnographic recording. The detection of plasma, urine, or salivary melatonin secretion is warranted to diagnose sleep-wake rhythm disorders in this specific population, but still remains a diagnostic tool used for research purpose. A diagnostic algorithm to asses sleep problems has been already described in children with ASD (Miano and Ferri 2010). After a detailed animalistic interview about sleep problems (sleep onset problems, many awakenings during sleep, presence of sleep hyperkinesias, myoclonic movements or stereotyped movements during sleep, many naps during daytime, daytime sleepiness, maturation of the sleep-wake rhythm, time of bedtime, and of final awakening in the morning), caregivers may fill sleep questionnaire, already used in children with ASD, such as the Children's Sleep Habits questionnaire or other validated sleep questionnaire (Bruni et al. 1997; Owens et al. 2000). In most of cases a behavioral insomnia and or circadian rhythm disorder is suspected. Sleep diaries and actigraphic recording of at least 1 week are warranted to confirm the diagnosis and assess sleep-wake behavior. Actigraphy provides useful information about sleep in the natural sleep environment variables. Collecting data representing body movement over time, actigraphy paints a picture of daily sleep-wake cycles, which can be useful in the diagnosis and evaluation of several clinical sleep disorders and treatment outcomes (Morgenthaler et al. 2007; Martin and Hakim 2011). Actigraphy is a simple device similar to a watch, usually worn in the nondominant wrist. The software calculates many sleep parameters such as total sleep time, sleep efficiency (defined as the percentage of time sleeping while in bed and lights off), and sleep latency (defined by time from lights off to sleep onset) and offers an overview of daytime activity, indirectly assessing daytime sleepiness and the number of naps (see Fig. 8.1, example of a sleep onset delayed insomnia recorded by actigraphy of a week). The sleep diary usually serves to ensure the functioning of actigraphy. On the contrary, when major sleep disorders are suspected, a video-polysomnographic recording (video PSG) with extensive EEG channels is warranted. Despite the sanitary cost, including the necessity of a sleep expert medical doctor for diagnosis, laboratory-attended video PSG-recording remains the gold standard for the pediatric diagnosis of nocturnal epilepsy, sleep disordered breathing, and sleep movements disorders (Aurora et al. 2011, 2012).

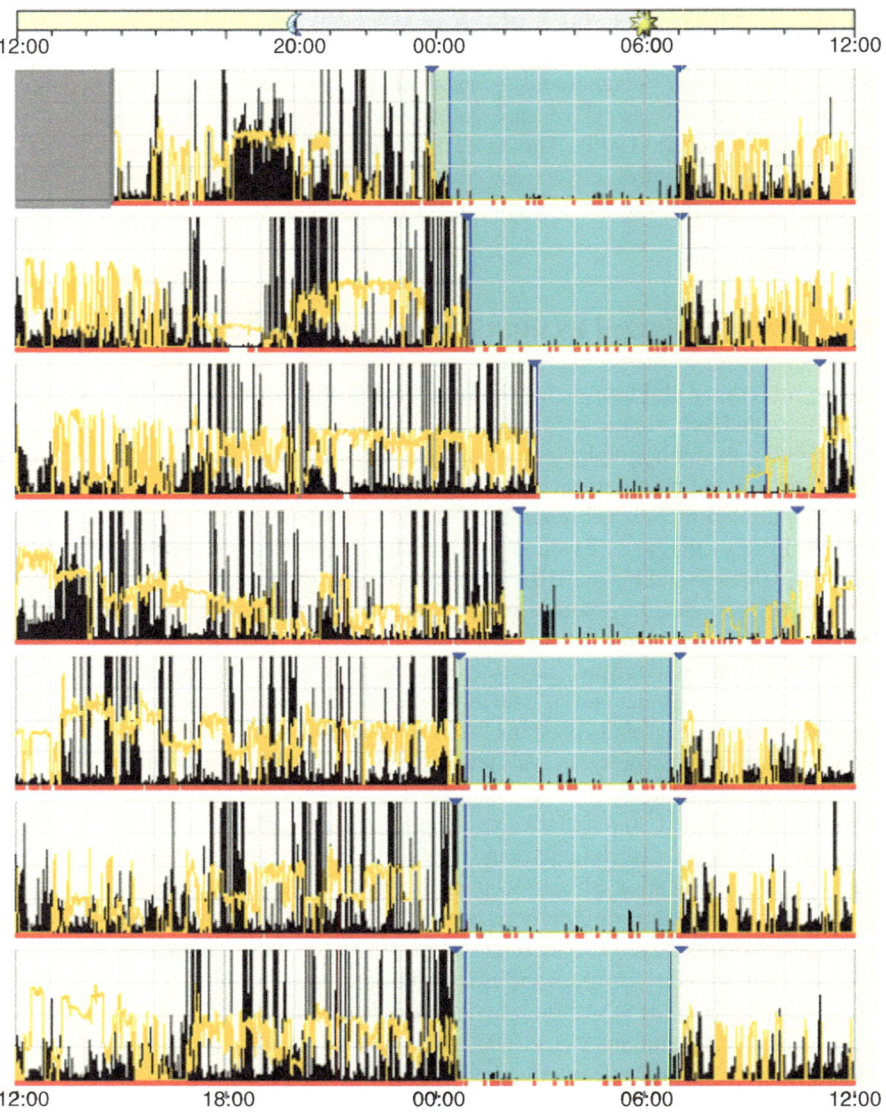

Fig. 8.1 An actigraphic recording of a week, showing a sleep onset delay with sleep onset after midnight (sleep period in *blue*)

The standard variables recorded during an overnight PSG recordings were at least eight EEG channels (frontal, central, temporal, and occipital monopolar montages referred to the contralateral mastoid or bilateral montages), according to the International "10–20" system to place electrodes in standardized scalp locations; an electrooculogram (electrodes placed 1 cm above the right outer cantus and 1 cm below the left outer cantus and referred to A1); and a submental electromyogram and an electrocardiogram (one derivation). Chest and abdominal movements and efforts and oronasal airflow are recorded with a thermocouple (or nasal pressure monitor when children tolerated a nasal cannula). Arterial oxygen saturation was monitored by means of a pulse oximeter. Recording usually starts at the patients' usual bedtime and continued until spontaneous awakening.

The following PSG variables are usually scored manually and automatically calculated, according to standard criteria (Berry et al. 2012a, b): time in bed (TIB), sleep period time (SPT; time from sleep onset to sleep end), total sleep time (TST; SPT minus time spent in wakefulness after sleep onset), sleep efficiency index (TST/TIB*100), sleep onset latency (SOL; time from lights out to sleep onset, defined as the first of two consecutive epochs of stage 1 sleep or one epoch of any other stage, in minutes), first rapid eye movement (REM) latency (FRL; time from sleep onset to the first REM epoch), minutes spent in each stage and percentage relative to SPT, number of stage shifts/hour, number of REM periods, number of awakenings/hour, percentage of each sleep stages (stage N1, N2, N3, REM sleep); central, obstructive, and mixed apnea events and the apnea hypopnea index (number of respiratory events during sleep), overnight oxygen saturation and desaturation index, leg movements (LMs), and periodic leg movements (PLMs) during sleep.

6   Neurobiological Bases and Genetic Overlap

Alterations of hormone secretion and neurotransmitters have been hypothesized for the pathogenesis of sleep disorders in ASD, such as abnormal dopaminergic activity in the low medial prefrontal cortex; high level of catecholamines in blood, urine, and CSF (Ernst et al. 1997); as well as abnormalities in the circadian secretion of melatonin. Recently mutations in circadian-relevant genes affecting gene function in ASD children have been reported, particularly two kinds of mutations that were detected only in individuals with ASD and sleep disorders (Yang et al. 2015). Melatonin is the "darkness hormone," involved in signaling the appropriate timing of the sleep and wake cycle. Melatonin regulates vigilance states: MT2 receptors are mainly involved in non-rapid eye movement sleep, whereas MT receptors are mainly involved in REM sleep. Melatonin has been shown to influence basal metabolism, oxidative stress, inflammation, and apoptosis and to prevent premature aging and tumorigenesis, and it seems to be critically involved in early development through its direct effects on placenta, developing neurons and glia, and its role in the ontogenetic establishment of diurnal rhythms (Tordjman et al. 2013).

Several studies have demonstrated abnormal melatonin regulation in individuals with autism compared with controls, including elevated daytime melatonin and significantly lower nocturnal melatonin (Ritvo et al. 1993; Nir et al. 1995; Kulman et al. 2000; Tordjman et al. 2005, 2012). More specifically abnormally low daytime and nighttime melatonin secretion was associated with an absence of melatonin circadian variation in some individuals with autism (Tordjman et al. 2012). Melke et al. (2008) found lower level of acetylserotonin O-methyltransferase (ASMT) activity, an enzyme which converts serotonin to melatonin, as well as genetic variation in the promoter of ASMT in children with ASD. Even though other studies failed to show a direct association of the promoter variants in ASMT with autism (Toma et al. 2007; Wang et al. 2013), genetic variation in ASMT has been reported to be more common in children with autism (Cai et al. 2008). More recently Veatch et al. (2015) demonstrated the alteration of two melatonin pathway genes in a subset of children with autism and sleep onset delay. A disruption of the serotonin-melatonin pathway with elevated whole-blood serotonin and decreased plasma melatonin has been also reported in 278 ASD patients and deficit of melatonin which is significantly associated with insomnia (Pagan et al. 2014). In contrast, a recent research showed relatively normal patterns of endogenous melatonin secretion during sleep (Goldman et al. 2014).

7   Treatment

The diagnosis of a sleep disorder is the first and the most important step in successful intervention. The identification and treatment of possible underlying medical, neurological, or psychiatric conditions should be part of a comprehensive, multidisciplinary approach to the treatment of children with ASD.

7.1   Nonmedical Treatment: Sleep Hygiene and Behavioral Interventions

Sleep hygiene and behavioral therapy are shown to be effective interventions for both typically developing children and for ASD children. Several studies have demonstrated effectiveness of behavioral interventions for bedtime problems, sleep onset, and sleep maintenance problems in children with ASD (Wiggs 2000; Thackeray 2002; Richdale and Wiggs 2005; Weiskop et al. 2005; Kuhn and Floress 2008). Thus, the first line of treatment in children with neurodevelopmental disabilities is to improve sleep hygiene, a set of sleep related behaviors which can promote a better sleep (Jan et al. 2008).

Basic principles of sleep hygiene include the selection of an appropriate bedtime, establishment of a positive consistent bedtime routine, and reduction of emotional and/or behavioral stimulation at night. As above stated, the association between media exposure, bedtime resistance, and sleep onset delay is strongly pronounced in ASD children; thus, minimizing television watching and playing computer or video games may represent an important intervention target for improving sleep (Engelhardt et al. 2013). Taking into consideration the night-to-night variability of sleep-wake patterns in children with ASD (Anders et al. 2011), it is equally important to pay attention to the consistency of the bedtime and risetime in the morning in order to enhance a regular sleep-wake cycle.

Furthermore, as previously stated, children with ASD frequently have hypersensitivity to environmental stimuli, including noises or tactile sensitivity to bedclothes or blankets. A parental survey conducted by Williams et al. (2006) indicated that wrapping a child in weighted blankets may be helpful in children with tactile sensitivities with sleep onset problems. More recently, Gringas et al. (2014) in a randomized placebo-controlled crossover design on 67 children with ASD reported that even though the use of a weighted blanket did not help for a longer period of time or to fall asleep faster or wake less often, as actigraphically demonstrated, it was favored by children and parents and was tolerated over the period.

The behavioral interventions used to treat insomnia in children with ASD are essentially the same as those used in typically developing children. Behavioral interventions can be utilized to set appropriate behavioral limits at bedtime and to promote the development of the more adaptive self-soothing skills (Williams et al. 2006). Among behavioral interventions, graduated extinction, where new behavior is taught in small steps, appears more appropriate when treating children with ASD (Wiggs 2000).

Despite promising evidence regarding the effectiveness of behavioral treatment in reducing settling problems and awakenings in children with ASD (Wiggs 2000; Thackeray 2002, Weiskop et al. 2005; Vriend et al. 2011), these interventions might be time intensive and expensive, particularly to support parents with face-to-face meeting (Montgomery et al. 2004). To partially overcome these problems, recently, Austin et al. (2013) evaluated the positive effect of a parent group program for children with ASD and sleep disturbances, which included workshop session as well as individualized treatment plans. More recently Malow (2014) evaluated the effect of individualized compared to group education sleep intervention on a large sample of 80 ASD children. Interestingly, mode of education did not differ in the positive effects of treatment. Moreover, Stuttard et al. (2015a) confirmed the efficacy of a group-delivered sleep management intervention for parents of children with intellectual disabilities including autism. In addition Stuttard et al. (2015b) in another pilot study demonstrated that it may be acceptable to support parents implementing a behavioral sleep intervention via telephone call. Even though this new approach seems to be effective, authors recommended flexibility when further face-to face contacts may be beneficial.

In ASD children with comorbid anxiety, family-based-cognitive-behavioral therapy displayed a significant reduction in frequency of sleep problems (Nadeau et al. 2014). In addition Papadopoulos et al. (2015) reported the efficacy of a brief sleep intervention in 28 school-aged children with ASD and comorbid ADHD. Children with ASD-ADHD reported not only a moderate to large improvement in sleep problems but also moderate improvement in quality of life.

7.2   Pharmacological Intervention

If a child fails to respond to sleep hygiene and behavioral intervention or has only partial response, pharmacological treatment options should be considered in conjunction with the ongoing behavioral therapy for sleep disorders.

There is growing evidence in particular for the use of melatonin. Melatonin is considered a nutritional supplement and is not regulated by the Food and Drug

Administration (FDA). Given this labeling, melatonin is readily available over the counter and relatively inexpensive. Several studies showed that exogenous melatonin is efficient in promoting sleep and is well tolerated, and no serious long-term adverse effects have been described (Jan et al. 1994; Dodge and Wilson 2001; Ross et al. 2002; Phillips and Appleton 2004; Gringas et al. 2012).

There have been relatively few trials utilizing melatonin exclusively in children with ASD. In an open-label trial, 15 children with Asperger's syndrome were administered 3 mg of immediate-release melatonin 30 min prior to bedtime for 2 weeks (Paavonen et al. 2003). Sleep latency decreased significantly from 40 to 21 min during treatment as measured by actigraphy. A second open-label study of children with autism utilized combined immediate- and controlled-release melatonin in a dose range of 3–6 mg (Giannotti et al. 2006). All of the children improved according to sleep diaries and questionnaires. A randomized, placebo-controlled trial of melatonin 5 mg was found effective in children with ASD and insomnia (Garstang and Wallis 2006). A larger retrospective study of over 100 children with ASD treated with melatonin documented minimal adverse effects, with improved sleep in 85 % of children treated (Andersen et al. 2008). A study on 24 ASD children with sleep onset delay using dose escalation of controlled-release melatonin, from 2 to 9 mg when clinically required, reported significant improvement in sleep latency within the first week of treatment (Malow et al. 2011). Furthermore, in a randomized double-blind crossover trial on 22 ASD children with sleep insomnia, Wright et al. (2011) reported significant improvement in sleep latency and total sleep time, as reported by parents in the melatonin group. Moreover, a randomized placebo-controlled study demonstrated the superior efficacy of the combination of controlled-release melatonin treatment with behavioral interventions in 134 children with autism and long-lasting sleep problems (Cortesi et al. 2012). In addition, four meta-analysis studies confirmed the beneficial effects of melatonin on sleep in ASD children with no or minus side effects (Guénolé et al. 2011; Doyen et al. 2011; Rossignol et al. 2011; Reading 2012).

There are likely several mechanisms by which melatonin may promote sleep in people with ASD. Melatonin may simply act as a hypnotic to promote sleep especially at higher than physiologic doses (Heuvel et al. 2005). When used as a hypnotic for sleep onset insomnia, melatonin should be given approximately 30 min prior to the desired bedtime. Melatonin also has a chronobiotic (phase-shifting) effect and therefore may be more effective in individuals with a delayed sleep phase when given several hours before bedtime. A dosage range of 1–3 mg is usually adequate, but on occasion, doses of 6 mg or higher are needed. Recently, Ayyash et al. (2015) demonstrated that increasing melatonin above 6 mg/night adds further benefit only in a small percentage of children with neurodevelopmental disabilities including autism. Liquid formulations are available and useful in children who have difficulty swallowing tablets. Extended-release melatonin may be helpful for the child with sleep maintenance difficulties (Jan et al. 2000; Giannotti et al. 2006; Cortesi et al. 2012). Once the sleep schedule stabilizes over several months, attempts should be made to discontinue melatonin.

Recently a positive effect of ramelteon, a selective melatonin receptor agonist, has been reported in three ASD children with circadian sleep disorders (Kawabe et al. 2014). Ramelteon is a relative new drug with high selectivity for the melatonin MT1 and MT2 receptors, which are located in the suprachiasmatic nucleus and have been implicated in the regulation of sleep-wake cycle. Authors reported that ramelteon reduce not only sleep disorders but autistic behavior as well.

There is limited research on the use of prescription medications with sedative properties for children with autism. One study demonstrated effectiveness of Niaprazine, a histamine H1-receptor antagonist with sedative properties which were available in Europe in treating insomnia in this population (Rossi et al. 1999). A recent retrospective study found that clonidine, an alpha-2 adrenergic receptor agonist, was effective in reducing sleep initiation latency and night awakening (Ming et al. 2008).

Successful pharmacological treatment of comorbid psychiatric disorders like ADHD, mood, and/or anxiety disorders as well as neurological conditions like epilepsy and movement disorders may help to alleviate symptoms of insomnia and markedly improve outcome.

Providing safety is the priority when treating parasomnias. Arousal disorders such as sleep terrors and sleep walking may be severe enough in children or adolescents to warrant pharmacotherapy. Clonazepam or tript-oh is the treatment of choice when a medication is indicated. Clonazepam is also effective in treating rhythmic movement disorder when the potential for injury is present as well as REM sleep behavior disorder also responds to clonazepam, although dopaminergic agents and melatonin have also been tried (Diomedi et al. 1999).

8 Discussion and Future Directions

The restoration of some basic regular physiological rhythms such as circadian rhythms may open new therapeutic perspectives in ASD. Both pharmacologic and behavioral interventions have demonstrated to be effective for the treatment of sleep problems in autistic children.

The most common types of behavioral interventions are unmodified extinction and various forms of graduated extinction, while melatonin has shown promising results restoring the impaired circadian melatonin rhythm in ASD. The synchronization of internal biological clocks may directly impact and improve social communication, stereotyped behaviors, and adaptation to environmental changes. Even though the results of controlled studies are limited, there are more data demonstrating the safety and effectiveness of melatonin in ASD than for other sedative/hypnotic drugs. We firmly suggest dual treatment for insomnia in ASD consisting of melatonin administration associated with behavioral intervention. Randomized clinical trials in ASD are warranted to establish potential therapeutic efficacy of melatonin for social communication impairments and stereotyped behaviors or interests (Tordjman et al. 2013).

References

International classification of sleep disorders (2014) 3rd edn. American Academy of Sleep Medicine, Darien

Accardo JA, Malow BA (2014) Sleep, epilepsy, and autism. Epilepsy Behav. pii: S1525-5050(14)00533-2

Anders TF et al (2011) Six month sleep-wake organization in pre-school-age children with developmental delay and typical development. Behav Sleep Med 829:92–106

Andersen IM et al (2008) Melatonin for insomnia in children with autism spectrum disorders. J Child Neurol 23:482–485

Association AP (1980) Diagnostic and statistical manual of mental disorders, 5th edn. American Psychiatric Association, Washington, DC, p 2013

Aurora RN, American Academy of Sleep Medicine et al (2011) Practice parameters for the respiratory indications for polysomnography in children. Sleep 34:379–388

Aurora RN et al (2012) Practice parameters for the non-respiratory indications for polysomnography and multiple sleep latency testing for children. Sleep 35:1467–1473

Austin et al (2013) Preliminary evaluation of stepwise program for children with sleep disturbance and developmental delay. Child Fam Behav Ther 35:195–211

Ayyash HF et al (2015) Melatonin for sleep disturbance in children with neurodevelopmental disorders: prospective observational naturalistic study. Expert Rev Neurother 4:1–7

Berry R, et al. for the American Academy of Sleep Medicine (2012a) The AASM manual for the scoring of sleep and associated events: rules, terminology and technical specifications. Darien: American Academy of Sleep Medicine. Version 2.0. www.aasmnet.org.

Berry RB, et al (2012b) Rules for scoring respiratory events in sleep: update of the 2007 AASM manual for the scoring of sleep and associated Events. Deliberations of the sleep apnea definitions task force of the American Academy of Sleep Medicine. J Clin Sleep Med 8:597–619

Bradley EA et al (2004) Comparing rates of psychiatric and behavior disorders in adolescents and young adults with severe intellectual disability with and without autism. J Autism Dev Disord 34:151–161

Bruni O et al (1997) Prevalence of sleep disorders in childhood and adolescence with headache: a case-control study. Cephalalgia 17:492–498

Cai G et al (2008) Multiplex ligation-dependent probe amplification for genetic screening in autism spectrum disorders: efficient identification of known microduplications and identification of a novel microduplication in ASMT. BMC Med Genomics I:50

Chantiluke K et al (2014) Disorder-specific functional abnormalities during temporal discounting in youth with Attention Deficit Hyperactivity Disorder (ADHD), autism and comorbid ADHD and autism. Psychiatry Res 223:113–120

Chez MG et al (2006) Frequency of epileptiform EEG abnormalities in a sequential screening of autistic patients with no known clinical epilepsy from 1996 to 2005. Epilepsy Behav 8:267–271

Clarke DF, Roberts W (2005) The prevalence of autistic spectrum disorder in children surveyed in a tertiary care epilepsy clinic. Epilepsia 46:1970–1977

Cohen S et al (2014) The relationship between sleep and behavior in autism spectrum disorder ASD: a review. J Neurodev Disord 6:44

Cortesi F et al (2010) Sleep in children with autism spectrum disorders. Sleep Med 11:659–664

Cortesi F et al (2012) Controlled-release melatonin, singly and combined with cognitive behavioral therapy for persistent insomnia in children with autism spectrum disorders: a randomized placebo-controlled trial. Sleep Res 21:700–709

Couturier JL et al (2005) Parental perception of sleep problems in children of normal intelligence with pervasive developmental disorders: prevalence, severity, and pattern. J Am Acad Child Adolesc Psychiatry 44:815–822

Delahaye J et al (2014) The relationship between health-related quality of life and sleep problems in children with autism spectrum disorders. Res Autism Spectr Disord 8:292–303

Diomedi M, Curatolo P, Scalise A, Placidi F, Caretto F, Gigli GL (1999) Sleep abnormalities in mentally retarded autistic subjects: Down's syndrome with mental retardation and normal subjects. Brain Dev 21(8):548–53

Dodge NN, Wilson GA (2001) Melatonin for treatment of sleep disorders in children with developmental disabilities. J Child Neurol 16:581–584

Doo S, Wing YK (2006) Sleep problems of children with pervasive developmental disorder: correlation with parental stress. Dev Med Child Neurol 48:650–655

Dosman CF et al (2007) Children with autism: effect of iron supplementation on sleep and ferritin. Pediatr Neurol 36:152–158

Doyen C et al (2011) Melatonin in children with autism spectrum disorders: recent and practical data. Eur Child Adolesc Psychiatry 20:231–239

Elrod MG, Hoods BS (2015) Sleep differences among children with autism spectrum disorders and typically developing peers: a meta-analysis. J Dev Behav Pediatr 36:166–177

Engelhardt CR et al (2013) Media use and sleep among boys with autism spectrum disorders, ADHD, or typical development. Pediatrics 132:1081–1089

Ernst M et al (1997) Low medial prefrontal dopaminergic activity in autistic children. Lancet 350, Erratum in: Lancet 1998; 351:454

Garstang J, Wallis M (2006) Randomized controlled trial of melatonin for children with autistic spectrum disorders and sleep problems. Child Care Health Dev 32:585–589

Giannotti F, Cortesi F, Cerquiglini A, Bernabei P (2006) An open-label study of controlled-release melatonin in treatment of sleep disorders in children with autism. J Autism Dev Disord 36(6):741–752

Giannotti F et al (2008) An investigation of sleep characteristics, EEG abnormalities and epilepsy of developmentally regressed and non-regressed autistic children. J Autism Dev Disord 38:1888–1897

Giannotti F et al (2011) Sleep in children with autism with and without developmental regression. J Sleep Res 20:338–347

Goldman SE et al (2014) Melatonin in children with autism spectrum disorders: endogenous and pharmacokinetic profiles in relation to sleep. J Autism Dev Disord 44:2525–2535

Goodlin-Jones BL et al (2008) Sleep patterns in preschool-age children with autism, developmental delay and typical development. J Am Acad Child Adolesc Psychiatry 47:930–938

Gringas P et al (2012) Melatonin for sleep problems in children with neurodevelopmental disorders: randomized double masked placebo controlled trial. Br Med J 345:1–16

Gringas P et al (2014) Weighted blankets and Sleep in Autistic children – a randomized controlled trial. Pediatrics 134:298–306

Guénolé F et al (2011) Melatonin for disordered sleep in individual with autism spectrum disorders: a systematic review and discussion. Sleep Med Rev 15:379–387

Heuvel CJ et al (2005) Melatonin as a hypnotic: con. Sleep Med Rev 9:71–80

Hodge D et al (2014) Sleep patterns in children with and without autism spectrum disorders: developmental comparisons. Res Dev Disabil 35:1631–1638

Hollway AJ et al (2011) Sleep correlates of pervasive developmental disorders: a review of the literature. Res Dev Disabil 32:1399–1421

Ivanenko A, Johnson K (2008) Sleep disturbances in children with psychiatric disorders. Semin Pediatr Neurol 15:70–78

Jan JE et al (1994) The treatment of sleep disorders with melatonin. Dev Med Child Neurol 36:97–107

Jan JE et al (2000) Clinical trials of controlled-release melatonin in children with sleep-wake cycle disorders. J Pineal Res 29:34–39

Jan JE et al (2008) Sleep hygiene for children with neurodevelopmental disabilities. Pediatrics 122:1343–1350

Johnson DA (2005) Gastroesophageal reflux disease and sleep disorders: a wake-up call for physicians and their patients. Rev Gastroenterol Disord 5(suppl 2):S3–S11

Johnson KP, Malow BA (2008) Sleep in children with autism spectrum disorders. Curr Neurol Neurosci Rep 8:155–161

Kawabe K et al (2014) The melatonin receptor agonist ramelteon effectively treats insomnia and behavioral symptoms in autistic disorders. Case Rep Psychiatry 2014:561071

Kotagal S, Broomall E (2012) Sleep in children with autism spectrum disorders. Pediatr Neurol 47:242–251

Krakowiak P et al (2008) Sleep problems in children with autism spectrum disorders, developmental delays, and typical development: a population-based study. J Sleep Res 17:197–206

Kuhn BR, Floress MT (2008) Nonpharmacological interventions for sleep disorders in children. In: Ivanenko A (ed) Sleep and psychiatric disorders in children and adolescents. Informa Healthcare, New York, pp 261–278

Kulman G et al (2000) Evidence of pineal endocrine hypofunction in autistic children. Neuroendocrinol Lett 20:31–34

Lewine JD et al (1999) Magnetoencephalographic patterns of epileptiform activity in children with regressive autism spectrum disorders. Pediatrics 104(3 Pt 1):405–418

Liu X et al (2006) Sleep disturbances and correlates of children with autism spectrum disorders. Child Psychiatry Hum Dev 37:179–191

Malow BA (2006) Searching for autism symptomatology in children with epilepsy – a new approach to an established comorbidity. Epilepsy Curr 6:150–152

Malow B (2014) A parent-based sleep education for children with autism spectrum disorders. J Autism Dev Disord 44:216–228

Malow BA, Mc Grew SG (2008) Sleep disturbance and autism. Sleep Med Clin 3:479–488

Malow BA et al (2006a) Characterizing sleep in children with autism spectrum disorders: a multidimensional approach. Sleep 29:1563–1571

Malow BA et al (2006b) Sleep and autism spectrum disorders. In: Tuchman R, Rapin I (eds) Autism: a neurological disorders of early brain development. Mac Keith Press, London, pp 188–201

Malow B et al (2011) Melatonin for sleep in children with autism: a controlled trial examining dose, tolerability and outcomes. J Autism Dev Disord 42:1729–1732

Martin JL, Hakim AD (2011) Wrist actigraphy. Chest 139:1514–1527

Matsuura H et al (2008) Dynamical properties of the two-process model for sleep-wake cycles in infantile autism. Cogn Neurodyn 2:221–228

May T et al (2015) Sleep in high functioning children with autism: Longitudinal developmental change and associations with behavior problems. Sleep Med 13:2–18

Mazurek MO et al (2015) Sleep problems in children with autism spectrum disorder: examining the contributions of sensory over-responsivity and anxiety. Sleep Med 16:270–279

Melke J et al (2008) Abnormal melatonin synthesis in autism spectrum disorders. Mol Psychiatry 13:90–98

Miano S, Ferri R (2010) Epidemiology and management of insomnia in children with autistic spectrum disorders. Paediatr Drugs 12:75–84

Miano S, Peraita-Adrados R (2014) Pediatric insomnia: clinical, diagnosis, and treatment. Rev Neurol 58:35–42

Miano S et al (2007) Sleep in children with autistic spectrum disorder: a questionnaire and polysomnographic study. Sleep Med 9:64–70

Miano S et al (2013) Case reports of sleep phenotypes of ADHD: from hypothesis to clinical practice. J Atten Disord 17:565–573

Ming X et al (2008) Autism spectrum disorders: concurrent clinical disorders. J Child Neurol 23:6–13

Montgomery P et al (2004) The relative efficacy of two brief treatments for sleep problems in young learning disabled children: a randomized controlled trial. Arch Dis Child 89:125–130

Morgenthaler T, Standards of Practice Committee, American Academy of Sleep Medicine et al (2007) Practice parameters for the use of actigraphy in the assessment of sleep and sleep disorders: an update for 2007. Sleep 30:519–529

Nadeau JM et al (2014) Frequency and clinical correlates of sleep-related problems among anxious youth with autism spectrum disorders. Child Psychiatry Hum Dev 46:558–566

Nally B et al (2000) Researchers in brief: the management of television and video by parents of children with autism. Autism 4:331–337

Nir I et al (1995) Brief report: circadian melatonin, thyroid-stimulating hormone, prolactin, and cortisol levels in serum of young adults with autism. J Autism Dev Disord 25:641–654

Owens JA et al (2000) The Children's Sleep Habits Questionnaire (CSHQ): psychometric properties of a survey instrument for school-aged children. Sleep 23:1043–1051

Owens JA et al (2010) Use of pharmacotherapy for insomnia in child psychiatry practice: a national survey. Sleep Med 11:692–700

Paavonen EJ et al (2003) Effectiveness of melatonin in the treatment of sleep disturbances in children with Asperger disorder. J Child Adolesc Psychopharmacol 13:83–95

Pagan C et al (2014) The serotonin-N acetylserotonin-melatonin pathway as a biomarker for autism spectrum disorders. Transl Psychiatry 4, e479, 1–8

Papadopoulos N et al (2015) The efficacy of a brief behavioral sleep intervention in school-aged children with ADHD and comorbid autism spectrum disorders. J Atten Disord. pii: 1087054714568565

Patzold LM et al (1998) An investigation into sleep characteristics of children with autism and Asperger's disorder. J Paediatr Child Health 34:528–533

Phillips L, Appleton R (2004) Systematic review of melatonin treatment in children with neurodevelopmental disabilities and sleep impairment. Dev Med Child Neurol 46:771–775

Polimeni MA et al (2005) A survey of sleep problems in autism, Asperger's disorder and typically developing children. J Intellect Dis Res 49:260–268

Reading R (2012) Melatonin in autism spectrum disorders: a systematic review and metanalysis. Child Care Health Dev 38:301–302

Richdale AL, Prior MR (1995) The sleep/wake rhythm in children with autism. Eur Child Adolesc Psychiatry 4:175–186

Richdale AL, Schreck KA (2009) Sleep problems in autism spectrum disorders: prevalence, nature and possible biopsychosocial etiologies. Sleep Med Rev. doi:10.1016/j.smrv.2009.02.003

Richdale A, Wiggs L (2005) Behavioral approaches to the treatment of sleep problems in children with developmental disorders. What is the state of the art? Int J Behav Consult Ther 1:165–189

Richdale AL et al (2014) The role of insomnia, pre-sleep arousal and psychopathology symptoms in daytime impairment in adolescents with high-functioning autism spectrum disorder. Sleep Med 15:1082–1088

Ritvo ER et al (1993) Elevated daytime melatonin concentrations in autism: a pilot study. Eur Child ASDolesc Psychiatry 2:75–78

Robinson AM, Richdale AL (2004) Sleep problems in children with an intellectual disabilities: parental perception of sleep problems and views of treatment effectiveness. Child Care, Health Dev 30:139–150

Rocca FL et al (2015) Narcolepsy during childhood: an update. Neuropediatrics 46:181–198

Rommelse NNJ et al (2011) A review on cognitive and brain endophenotypes that may be common in autism spectrum disorder and attention-deficit/hyperactivity disorder and facilitate the search for pleiotropic genes. Neurosci Biobehav Rev 35:1363–1396

Ross C et al (2002) Melatonin treatment for sleep disorders in children with neurodevelopmental disorders: an observational study. Dev Med Child Neurol 44:339–344

Rossi PG et al (1999) Niaprazine in the treatment of autistic disorder. J Child Neurol 14:547–550

Rossignol DA et al (2011) Melatonin in autism spectrum disorders: a systematic review and metanalysis. Dev Med Child Neurol 53:783–792

Schreck KA, Mulick JA (2000) Parental report of sleep problems in children with autism. J Autism Dev Disord 30:127–135

Stuttard L et al (2015a) Replacing home visits with telephone calls to support parents implementing a sleep management intervention: findings from a pilot study and implications for future research. Child Care Health Dev 41:1074–1081

Stuttard L et al (2015b) A preliminary investigation into the effectiveness of a group-delivered sleep management for parents of children with intellectual disabilities. J Int Dis 19:342–355

Thackeray EJ, Richdale AL (2002) The behavioural treatment of sleep difficulties in children with intellectual disabilities. Behav Interv 17:211–231

Thirumalai SS et al (2002) Rapid eye movement sleep behavior disorder in children with autism. J Child Neurol 17:173–178

Toma CF et al (2007) Is ASMT a susceptibility gene for autism spectrum disorders? A replication study in European populations. Mol Psychiatry 12:977–979

Tordjman S et al (2005) Nocturnal excretion of 6-sulphatoxymelatonin in children and adolescents with autistic disorder. Biol Psychiatry 57:134–138

Tordjman S et al (2012) Day and nighttime excretion of 6-sulphatoxymelatonin in adolescents and young adults with autistic disorder. Psychoneurocrinology 37:1990–1997

Tordjman S et al (2013) Advances in the research of melatonin in autism spectrum disorders: literature review and new perspectives. Int J Mol Sci 14:20508–20542

Tordjman S et al (2014) Altered circadian patterns of salivary cortisol in low-functioning children and adolescents with autism. Psychoneurocrinology 50:227–245

Tordjman S et al (2015) Autism as a disorder of biological and behavioral rhythms: toward new therapeutic perspectives. Front Pediatr 3:1

Valdizán-Usón JR et al (2002) Nocturnal polysomnogram in childhood autism without epilepsy. Rev Neurol 34:1101–1105

Veatch OJ et al (2015) Genetic variation in melatonin pathway enzymes in children with autism spectrum disorder and comorbid sleep onset delay. J Autism Dev Disord 45:100–110

Vriend JL et al (2011) Behavioral interventions for sleep problems in children with autism spectrum disorders: current findings and future directions. J Pediatr Psychol 36:1017–1029

Wang L et al (2013) Sequencing ASMT identifies rare mutations in Chinese Han patients with autism. PLoS One 8:e 53727

Weiskop S et al (2005) Behavioral treatment to reduce sleep problems in children with autism or fragile X syndrome. Dev Med Child Neurol 47:94–104

Wiggs L (2001) Sleep problems in children with developmental disorders. J R Soc Med 94:177–179

Wiggs L, France K (2000) Behavioural treatments for sleep problems in children and adolescents with physical illness, psychological problems or intellectual disabilities. Sleep Med Rev 4:299–314

Wiggs L, Stores G (2004) Sleep patterns and sleep disorders in children with autistic spectrum disorders: insights using parent report and actigraphy. Dev Med Child Neurol 46:372–380

Williams G et al (2006) Parent perceptions of efficacy for strategies used to facilitate sleep in children with autism. J Dev Phys Disabil 18:25–33

Wright B et al (2011) Melatonin versus placebo in children with autism spectrum conditions and severe sleep problems not amenable to behavior, management strategies: a randomized controlled crossover trial. J Autism Dev Disord 41:175–184

Yang et al (2015) Circadian-relevant genes are highly polymorphic in autism spectrum disorder patients Brain Dev (in press)

Personality Disorders and Autism Spectrum Disorder: What Is Similar and What Is Different?

Kathrin Sevecke, Luise Poustka, and Christian Popow

1   Introduction

Personality disorders (PDs) are mental disorders characterized by enduring maladaptive patterns of cognition and behavior, causing difficulties in personal and social functioning (American Psychiatric Association 2013). The origins of PDs are poorly understood; recent pathogenic models are based on traumatic negative (early) childhood experiences and on genetic background (Ballard et al. 2015; Chanen and Kaess 2012). In contrast to personality, i.e., mental traits that characterize human beings, PDs are associated with significant dysfunctional experience and behavior, a number of comorbid conditions, and severe personal disadvantages. These endanger personal well-being, education, social and occupational integration, and relationships (Biskin 2015).

Autism spectrum disorder (ASD) is a heterogeneous group of pervasive disorders characterized by problems of social communication and interaction, restrictive interests, and repetitive behaviors (American Psychiatric Association 2013). Caused by genetic deficiencies that impair brain networking, ASD shows a broad range of severity of impaired intellectual functioning, inflexibility, and personal and social dysfunction. There are multiple comorbid conditions, e.g., concerning sensory integration, attention, neurology, anxiety, and PDs. ASD are not curable, but improvements of development and personal and social functioning may be attained through

K. Sevecke (✉)
Department of Child and Adolescent Psychiatry, Innsbruck Medical University,
Innsbruck, Austria
e-mail: kathrin.sevecke@tirol-kliniken.at

L. Poustka • C. Popow
Department of Child and Adolescent Psychiatry, Vienna Medical University, Vienna, Austria
e-mail: Luise.Poustka@meduniwien.at

© Springer International Publishing Switzerland 2016   129
L. Mazzone, B. Vitiello (eds.), *Psychiatric Symptoms and Comorbidities in Autism Spectrum Disorder*, DOI 10.1007/978-3-319-29695-1_9

structured therapy for low-functioning children and through appropriate psychological and pharmacological therapy for higher-functioning children and adolescents. In this paper, we will focus on ASD patients with normal intellectual capacity; the relationships between low-functioning ASD patients and PDs have not yet been explored.

The relationships and overlapping psychopathology between ASD and PDs, although evident (especially for clusters A and C), are only poorly described and understood. These areas of overlap include pervasive impairment, abnormal development, stable patterns, long duration, onset in childhood to adolescence or early adulthood, and social impairment (Miller and Ozonoff 1997). However, a PD should be excluded "if the enduring pattern is not better accounted for as a manifestation or consequence of any other mental disorder" (American Psychiatric Association 2013). In this article, we will focus on these complex relationships, drawing upon available literature and aiming to contribute to the knowledge and (medical) handling of both disorders. We will especially focus on prevalence, phenomenology and clinical issues, common and uncommon features of PDs and ASD, and assessment and treatment.

2   Prevalence

PDs are among the most prevalent disorders in adulthood, reaching rates of 10% in community samples (Coid et al. 2006) and up to 50% in clinical samples (American Psychiatric Association 2000; Sevecke and Krischer 2008). Longitudinal studies suggest that prevalence rates of PDs are higher in adolescence and decline linearly up to the age of 27 (Chanen and Kaess 2012). Differences in prevalence rates may be explained by nonuniform interpretation of diagnostic criteria and the various classification systems.

The diagnosis of a PD is less stable than formerly expected (Biskin 2015; Skodol et al. 2005; Stepp 2012) and differs among the various types. PD traits such as "self-injurious behavior" are less stable than states such as "affective instability" and "impulsivity." Symptom stability is relatively stable over time for borderline (BPD), histrionic, and schizotypal PD and less stable for other categorical diagnoses.

3   Phenomenology, Comorbidity, and Clinical Issues

PD types are differently described by the various diagnostic systems: ICD-10 lists eight categories and a number of "others"; DSM-IV defined three clusters (A: odd, B: dramatic, C: anxious) and ten PDs in a separate diagnostic axis; and DSM-5 created a hybrid model, defining six categories of core impairments (antisocial, avoidant, borderline, narcissistic, obsessive-compulsive, and schizotypal PD, Criterion A) and five high-order traits (negative emotionality, detachment, antagonism, disinhibition, psychoticism, Criterion B). This new model reflects the complexity of PDs, improves discriminant validity and stability of the diagnosis, reduces comorbidity, and allows for assessing personal (identity and self-directedness) and interpersonal (empathy and intimacy) functioning. Although personality traits may be present in early childhood, a definite PD diagnosis is now permitted in adolescence, respecting that early intervention and adequate psychological and pharmacological therapy may result in significant functional improvement and even cure. In so doing, therapeutic nihilism and the mischaracterization of PDs as lifelong conditions should be avoided.

Patients with an increased symptom level are more severely affected in their psychosocial functioning. A high level of cluster A symptoms has been related to lower educational levels and job performance (Cohen et al. 2005).

Diagnostic and statistical manual of mental disorders- Fifth edition (DSM-5) has also introduced revised specifications for ASD: ASD is now a spectrum disorder, with two main symptoms – (1) deficits in social communication and interaction and (2) restricted interests and repetitive behavior. The previous categories no longer exist. Moreover, DSM-5 has introduced specifiers, intellectual and language impairment, association with a known medical or genetic condition, and three severity levels.

PDs and ASD share many comorbid conditions that aggravate the severity of the disorders. Comorbidities of BPD mainly relate to attention deficit (ADHD), mood, anxiety, posttraumatic stress disorder (PTSD), and eating disorders (EDs). The close relationship between antisocial PD (ASPD) and ADHD remains stable into adulthood (Mannuzza et al. 1998; Nigg et al. 2002; Rösler et al. 2008; Sevecke and Krischer 2008). In addition, characteristics of ASPD, BPD, and early complex PTSD and problems of interaction may overlap (Brunner et al. 2001; Schmid et al. 2010), and there are close similarities between PTSD and BPD (Jucksch et al. 2009; Krischer and Sevecke 2008). Comorbidities of ASD mainly relate to ADHD and sensory integration problems and mood, tic, and anxiety disorders.

There are only a few studies relating PS and ASD. Generally, adolescents and adults with PDs and ASD face problems in social interaction, mentalizing abilities, and building and maintaining stable relationships. Cluster A and C PDs seem to be more prevalent in ASD patients (Lugnegård et al. 2012), whereas ASD psychopathology seems to protect patients from cluster B PDs. This could be related to early difficulties and less interest in social interaction in ASD, limiting the effects of poor parenting and inconsistent parent-child interaction on the developing personality. Subjectively experienced excessive emotional demands leading to temper tantrums could be a link between ASD and cluster B PDs, but the backgrounds seem to be different: children with ASD are overburdened because of their limited cognitive flexibility, whereas BPD patients are overburdened by their difficulties in expressing and regulating their emotions (Jarnecke et al. 2015). Moreover, although BPD and ASD patients exhibit social problem-solving deficits, the former have intense but unstable social relationships and strive to avoid abandonment, whereas ASD patients seem to be socially more independent and to display less interest in social interactions (King-Casas and Chiu 2012). There is also a sex difference: ASD patients are predominantly male, while PDs show a female predominance.

Tantam (1988) and Esterberg et al. (2008) have described more severe current and past autistic features, such as social impairment and unusual interests and behavior in adolescents with schizotypal PD (SPD) compared to normal and other PD controls. Hurst et al. (2006), studying patients with Asperger's syndrome and SPD, found overlapping diagnostic criteria and correlations between social-interpersonal and communication-disorganized areas between the two disorders. Personality traits that are similar but less severe than in ASD are seen in the "broader autism phenotype" (BAP), comprising the traits "rigid," "impulsive," "aloof," "shy," "tactless," "reserved/schizoid," "irritable," "hypersensitive to criticism," "neurotic," "undemonstrative," and "anxious" (Sucksmith et al. 2011; Vannucchi et al. 2014).

Lugnegård et al. (2012), investigating 54 young adults with the clinical diagnosis of Asperger's syndrome (DSM-IV criteria, SKID-II interview), found marked PD symptoms in one-half of the autistic patients, two-thirds of the male, and one-third of the female population. The PD criteria were fulfilled for only four PDs, schizoid, schizotypal, avoidant, and obsessive-compulsive PD, and there were no cluster B diagnoses.

According to Hare and Neumann (2009), psychopathy as a specific PD sub-type and ASD are both associated with strong deficits in empathy. Empathy deficits differed, however, in both groups of patients in genetic, cognitive, and neurologic aspects (Wallace et al. 2012). Specifically, individuals with psychopathic personality traits had problems in processing emotional stimuli, had reduced levels of anxiety, and had deficits in ethical reasoning, whereas patients with ASD had difficulties with the cognitive processing of emotional cues (Rogers et al. 2006). Roberz et al. (2013) discuss the differential diagnosis in regard to a case report about a 17-year-old boy. ASD patients perceive the suffering of others as aversive (Blair 1999; Sigman et al. 2003). ASD patients also have difficulties understanding the reasoning and feeling of others and seem to act insensitively. Yet when information is presented in such a way that enables them to emotionally understand the problems of others, they feel and care empathically normal (Jones et al. 2010).

Anckarsater (2006) reviewed brain imaging similarities between ASD and aggressive PD or psychopathy, especially in regard to hypoactivity and structural reduction of the prefrontal cortex and the limbic circuitry. Patients with ASPD show smaller prefrontal and cingulate cortices (Yang et al. 2009), while ASD patients show volume reductions in the temporal and parietal areas (Scheel et al. 2011; Wallace et al. 2010, 2012).

Diagnostic evaluation for PDs includes semi-structured instruments such as SCID-II (Structured Clinical Interview for DSM-IV (First et al. 1997)) and IPDE (International Personality Disorder Examination (Loranger 1994)). The diagnosis of ASD relies on ADOS 2 (Autism Diagnostic Observation Schedule (Poustka et al. 2015)) and ADI-R (Autism Diagnostic Interview – Revised (Bölte et al. 2006)), both of which assess autistic symptoms in a semi-structured way. Patients with PD or ASD are not always aware of their clinical problems, and this leads to interpersonal difficulties. As patients may not report their problems, it is essential to also rely on external sources of information, such as parents, relatives, and teachers. Furthermore, experienced clinicians will detect interpersonal dysfunctions by analyzing transference and countertransference phenomena.

4   Treatment

4.1   Nonmedical Interventions

A number of effective psychotherapeutic programs and manuals for treating (B)PDs are available for adults. For adolescents, these therapies – with the exception of DBT-A – have not yet been fully evaluated:

- Specific psychodynamic therapies: Transference-Focused Psychotherapy (TFP (Clarkin et al. 2004)) and Mentalization-Based Treatment (MbT (Bateman and Fonagy 2006)) and Adolescent Identity Treatment (AIT (Foelsch et al. 2013))
- Specific cognitive behavioral therapies: Dialectical Behavior Therapy (DBT and DBT-A (Linehan 1993)) and Schema Therapy (Young et al. 2003)

Ongoing clinical trials for the treatment of adolescents with PDs aim to respect the specific needs of this age group (see overviews: Krischer et al. 2006; Krischer and Sevecke 2010). Examples of modified adult treatment protocols are Adolescent Identity Treatment (AIT (Foelsch et al. 2008)), Transference-Focused Psychotherapy for Adolescents (TFP-A (Fleischhaker et al. 2011)), and Dialectic Behavioral Therapy for Adolescents (DBT-A (Miller et al. 1997)). These therapies focus more on identity diffusion than on identity crisis (Foelsch et al. 2010). Identity diffusion entails the lack of an integrative self-concept, similarly lacking in regard to significant persons. Identity diffusion is a prerequisite for developing adolescent PDs. The patient describes himself or herself and others in a highly chaotic way, unable to detect or integrate contradictions (Clarkin et al. 2004). Adolescent PD therapy aims at improving interpersonal relationships with friends, parents, and teachers. It further aims at defining lifetime goals, developing a sense of self-worth, and achieving a stable identity.

4.2   Pharmacological Interventions

Pharmacological interventions for ASD and PDs are only symptomatic and supportive. The main target symptoms are aggressive behavior/temper tantrums, depression, sleep problems, and ADHD; in ASD patients with seizures, anticonvulsive medication is indicated. A recent field study on psychopharmacological treatment in Germany (Bachmann et al. 2013) included 1,124 patients, 0.5 % having the diagnosis of ASD. One-third of the ASD patients received medication, with methylphenidate and risperidone the most frequently prescribed substances. Pharmacological studies on treating PDs mainly focus on BPD (Paris 2011), with low evidence (Klar and Siever 1984). Treatment guidelines, e.g., for BPD (Oldham et al. 2001), are poorly evidence supported and are no longer up to date.

Neuroleptics are widely used to decrease intrapersonal stress levels, enabling a distancing from environmental stressors and a reduction of impulsivity and reactive aggressive behavior. Although widely used, neuroleptic treatment shows poor evidence of efficacy because large RCTs are lacking, especially for second-generation antipsychotics.

Anticonvulsants – aside from their use in epilepsy and bipolar disorder – are commonly used to reduce impulsivity and aggressive behavior. The evidence of such treatment is, however, poor (Huband et al. 2010).

Antidepressants are generally less effective in ASD (Williams et al. 2013) and PD (Paris 2011). This may be caused by the background and unchanging intrapersonal strain (due to flexibility problems) or by neuro-functional differences that are poorly understood.

The efficacy of ADHD medication, specifically methylphenidate and atomoxetine, has been proven in several prospective trials in ASD patients. Both medications seem to be less effective in ASD and PD patients than in normotypic and non-PD ADHD patients. However, methylphenidate (Simonoff et al. 2013) and atomoxetine (Handen et al. 2015) are effective in children with ASD, with atomoxetine showing a slightly better side effect profile. (B)PD patients with comorbid ADHD also benefit from these two medications (Newcorn et al. 2007). In addition, aggressive behavior (Blader et al. 2013) and the occurrence of SUD (Steinhausen and Bisgaard 2014) are reduced, and psychotherapeutic adherence improved with long-term medication (Prada et al. 2015).

5   Discussion and Future Directions

Clinical diagnosis and treatment of adolescents with PDs and ASD are sensitive, complex tasks that require specific knowledge and experience. The available diagnostic tools, mainly structured interviews and clinical observation, are relatively sensitive, specific, and reliable.

The findings to date and the abandoned age limitation for the assessment of PD (DSM-5) clearly justify the diagnosis of PDs in adolescence, but more work is necessary to better identify and understand age-specific processes and characteristics. Early, careful diagnosis of adolescents with PS, followed by specific treatment, is certainly indicated. It is noteworthy that large numbers of patients, when treated appropriately, are able to go into remission, rendering therapeutic nihilism as a consequence of presumed "incurability" unwarranted.

The new DSM-5 criteria for both groups of disorders provide a courageous approach, enhancing the quality of dimensional diagnosis. For PDs, abandoning the age limit of 18 and introducing a hybrid disorder model, keeping "old" categories and adding five high-order traits and 25 trait facets, will help characterizing the clinical picture more precisely. In ASD patients, emphasizing common problems, adding specifiers and severity levels, and abandoning categorization will likely increase diagnostic precision. Nevertheless, longitudinal studies for both groups of disorders are needed to better characterize the stability of the diagnostic criteria and the effects of specific therapies. For both groups of disorders, access to specific therapy and early, accurate diagnosis are essential to providing appropriate support.

As in all disorders, comorbidity is crucial for clinical severity, vocational success, and quality of life. The two disorders share multi-comorbid conditions, including ADHD and mood, anxiety, dysexecutive, and other disorders that further impair social functioning. Treatment must therefore consider the part of impairment caused by comorbid conditions.

The relationship between PDs and ASD is complex and not clearly defined. There are similarities, e.g., social ostracism, poor emotional control, comorbid conditions, unknown stability of symptoms, and therapy-related alleviation, as well as differences, e.g., age at onset, intellectual performance, social skills, and fears of abandonment. Some PDs and ASD and schizotypal PD show significant overlap. One of the main differences, besides age at onset, is etiology: ASD is primarily related to genetic problems of brain networks, with less parental impact, whereas PDs usually have a family and social background but are predominantly acquired disorders, related, for example, to poor parental functioning and repeated traumatization.

Nevertheless, PDs, especially those with schizotypal personality traits, and ASD share impaired social functioning due to emotional dysfunction. They appear to be of different etiology, however, which is apparent in their differing genetic, cognitive, and neuronal characteristics. The key point for differential diagnosis between PD and ASD thus appears to lie in the precise assessment of patients' empathy deficit.

Future work will likely focus on long-term epidemiology, etiology (genetics, inborn and acquired problems), and therapy. Precise diagnostics will influence specific therapies. The introduction of the dimensional-categorical hybrid model of the DSM-5, with its assessment of traits and trait facets, now allows for a better differentiation and characterization within personality pathology profiles. It may indeed also be helpful to create such profiles for patients with ASD.

Other questions concern social integration and specific vocational training as well as tailor-made and cost-effective psychotherapies for specific clinical entities. Similarly, the long-term effect of psychotherapies remains to be explored.

References

American Psychiatric Association (2000) Diagnostic and statistical manual of mental disorders, fourth edition, text revision (DSM-IV-TR). American Psychiatric Association, Washington, DC

American Psychiatric Association (2013) Diagnostic and statistical manual of mental disorders. Fifth edition (DSM-5). American Psychiatric Association, Arlington

Anckarsater H (2006) Central nervous changes in social dysfunction: autism, aggression, and psychopathy. Brain Res Bull 69(3):259–265. doi:10.1016/j.brainresbull.2006.01.008

Bachmann CJ, Manthey T, Kamp-Becker I, Glaeske G, Hoffmann F (2013) Psychopharmacological treatment in children and adolescents with autism spectrum disorders in Germany. Res Dev Disabil 34:2551–2563

Ballard ED, Van Eck K, Hart SR, Storr CL, Breslau N, Wilcox HC (2015) Latent classes of childhood trauma exposure predict the development of behavioral health outcomes in adolescence and young adulthood. Psychol Med 45(15):3305–3316

Bateman A, Fonagy P (2006) Mentalization-based treatment for borderline personality disorder. Oxford University Press, Oxford

Biskin RS (2015) The lifetime course of borderline personality disorder. Can J Psychiatry 60(7):303–308

Blader JC, Pliszka SR, Kafantaris V, Foley CA, Crowell JA, Carlson GA, . . . Daviss WB (2013) Callous-unemotional traits, proactive aggression, and treatment outcomes of aggressive children with attention-deficit/hyperactivity disorder. J Am Acad Child Adolesc Psychiatry 52(12): 1281–1293. doi:10.1016/j.jaac.2013.08.024

Blair RJR (1999) Psychophysiological responsiveness to the distress of others in children with autism. Personal Individ Differ 26(3):477–485. doi:10.1016/s0191-8869(98)00154-8

Bölte S, Rühl D, Schmötzer G, Poustka F (2006) ADI-R Diagnostisches Interview für Autismus - Revidiert Deutsche Fassung des Autism diagnostic interview – revised von Michael Rutter, Ann Le Couteur und Catherine Lord (1st ed). Huber/Hogrefe, Bern

Brunner R, Parzer P, Resch F (2001) Dissoziative Symptome und traumatische Lebensereignisse bei Jugendlichen mit einer Borderline-Störung. Persönlichkeitsstörungen 5:4–12

Chanen AM, Kaess M (2012) Developmental pathways to borderline personality disorder. Curr Psychiatry Rep 14(1):45–53. doi:10.1007/s11920-011-0242-y

Clarkin JF, Levy KN, Lenzenweger MF, Kernberg OF (2004) The Personality Disorders Institute/ Borderline Personality Disorder Research Foundation randomized control trial for borderline personality disorder: rationale, methods, and patient characteristics. J Personal Disord 18(1):52–72. doi:10.1521/pedi.18.1.52.32769

Cohen P, Crawford TN, Johnson JG, Kasen S (2005) The children in the community study of developmental course of personality disorder. J Personal Disord 19(5):131–140. doi:10.1521/pedi.2005.19.5.466

Coid J, Yang M, Tyrer P, Roberts A, Ullrich S (2006) Prevalence and correlates of personality disorder in Great Britain. Br J Psychiatry 188:423–431

Deutschsprachige Fassung der Autism Diagnostic Observation Schedule – 2 von C. Lord, M. Rutter, P.C. DiLavore, S. Risi, K. Gotham und S.L. Bishop (Module 1-4) und C. Lord, R.J. Luyster, K. Gotham und W. Guthrie (Kleinkind-Modul) (1st ed). Hogrefe, Bern

Esterberg ML, Trotman HD, Brasfield JL, Compton MT, Walker EF (2008) Childhood and current autistic features in adolescents with schizotypal personality disorder. Schizophr Res 104(1–3):265–273. doi:10.1016/j.schres.2008.04.029

First MB, Gibbon M, Spitzer RL, Williams JB (1997) Structured clinical interview for DSM-IV (SCID-I/SCID-II). American Psychiatric Publishers, Arlington

Fleischhaker C, Sixt B, Schulz E (2011) DBT-A Dialektisch-behaviorale Therapie für Jugendliche. Springer Science + Business Media, Berlin

Foelsch PA, Kernberg OF, Krischer MK (2008) Übertragungsfokussierte Psychotherapie für Jugendliche. Prax Kinderpsychol Kinderpsychiatr 57(8–9):662–692

Foelsch PA, Odom A, Arena H, Krischer MK, Sevecke K, Schlüter-Müller S (2010) Differenzierung zwischen Identitätskrise und Identitätsdiffusion und ihre Bedeutung für die Behandlung – am Beispiel einer Kasuistik. Praxis Kinderpsychologie Kinderpsychiatrie 59:418–434. doi:10.13109/prkk.2008.57.89.662

Foelsch P, Schlüter-Müller S, Odom A, Arena H, Borzutzky A, Schmeck K (2013) Behandlung von Jugendlichen mit Identitätsstörungen (AIT). Springer, Berlin

Handen BL, Aman MG, Arnold LE, Hyman SL, Tumuluru RV, Lecavalier L, . . . Smith T (2015) Atomoxetine, parent training, and their combination in children with autism spectrum disorder and attention-deficit/hyperactivity disorder. J Am Acad Child Adolesc Psychiatry 54(11):905–915. doi:10.1016/j.jaac.2015.08.013

Hare RD, Neumann CS (2009) Psychopathy: assessment and forensic implications. Can J Psychiatry 54(12):791–802. doi:10.1093/med/9780199551637.003.0007

Huband N, Ferriter M, Nathan R, Jones H (2010) Antiepileptics for aggression and associated impulsivity. Cochrane Database Syst Rev (2):CD003499. doi:10.1002/14651858.CD003499.pub3

Hurst RM, Nelson-Gray RO, Mitchell JT, Kwapil TR (2006) The relationship of Asperger's characteristics and Schizotypal personality traits in a non-clinical adult sample. J Autism Dev Disord 37(9):1711–1720. doi:10.1007/s10803-006-0302-z

Jarnecke AM, Miller ML, South SC (2015) Daily diary study of personality disorder traits: momentary affect and cognitive appraisals in response to stressful events. Personal Disord. doi:10.1037/per0000157

Jones AP, Happé FGE, Gilbert F, Burnett S, Viding E (2010) Feeling, caring, knowing: different types of empathy deficit in boys with psychopathic tendencies and autism spectrum disorder. J Child Psychol Psychiatry 51(11):1188–1197. doi:10.1111/j.1469-7610.2010.02280.x

Jucksch V, Salbach-Andrae H, Lehmkuhl U (2009) Persönlichkeitsentwicklung im Kindes- und Jugendalter. Nervenarzt 80(11):1322–1326. doi:10.1007/s00115-009-2805-2

King-Casas B, Chiu PH (2012) Understanding interpersonal function in psychiatric illness through multiplayer economic games. Biol Psychiatry 72(2):119–125. doi:10.1016/j.biopsych.2012.03.033

Klar H, Siever LJ (1984) The psychopharmacologic treatment of personality disorders. Psychiatr Clin North Am 7(4):791–801

Krischer MK, Sevecke K (2008) Early traumatization and psychopathy in female and male juvenile offenders. Int J Law Psychiatry 31(3):253–262. doi:10.1016/j.ijlp.2008.04.008

Krischer MK, Sevecke K (2010, July 1–3) The prevalence of personality disorders in adolescent in-patients. Paper presented at the 1st International Congress on Borderline Personality Disorders, Berlin

Krischer M, Sevecke K, Döpfner M, Lehmkuhl G (2006) Persönlichkeitsstörungsmerkmale im Kindes- und Jugendalter: Konzepte, methodische Ansätze und empirische Ergebnisse. Z Kinder Jugendpsychiatr 34(2):87–100. doi:10.1024/1422-4917.34.2.87

Linehan M (1993) Cognitive-behavioral treatment of borderline personality disorder, 1st edn. The Guilford Press, New York

Loranger AW (1994) The international personality disorder examination. Arch Gen Psychiatry 51(3):215–224. doi:10.1001/archpsyc.1994.03950030051005

Lugnegård T, Hallerbäck MU, Gillberg C (2012) Personality disorders and autism spectrum disorders: what are the connections? Compr Psychiatry 53(4):333–340. doi:10.1016/j.comppsych.2011.05.014

Mannuzza S, Klein RG, Bessler A, Malloy P, LaPadula M (1998) Adult psychiatric status of hyperactive boys grown up. Am J Psychiatry 155(4):493–498. doi:10.1176/ajp.155.4.493

Miller JN, Ozonoff S (1997) Did Asperger's cases have Asperger disorder? A research note. J Child Psychol Psychiatry 38(2):247–251

Miller AL, Rathus JH, Linehan MM, Wetzler S, Leigh E (1997) Dialectical behavior therapy adapted for suicidal adolescents. J Psychiatr Pract 3(2):78–86. doi:10.1097/00131746-199703000-00002

Newcorn JH, Weiss M, Stein MA (2007) The complexity of ADHD: diagnosis and treatment of the adult patient with comorbidities. CNS Spectr 12(8 Suppl 12):1–14, quiz 15–16

Nigg JT, John OP, Blaskey LG, Huang-Pollock CL, Willicut EG, Hinshaw SP, Pennington B (2002) Big five dimensions and ADHD symptoms: links between personality traits and clinical symptoms. J Personal Soc Psychol 83(2):451–469. doi:10.1037/0022-3514.83.2.451

Oldham JM, Gabbard GO, Goin MK, Gunderson J, Soloff P, Spiegel D, . . . Phillips KA (2001) Practice guideline for the treatment of patients with borderline personality disorder. J Psychiatry 1–82

Paris J (2011) Pharmacological treatments for personality disorders. Int Rev Psychiatry 23(3):303–309. doi:10.3109/09540261.2011.586993

Poustka L, Rühl D, Feineis-Matthews S, Bölte S, Poustka F, Hartung M (2015) Diagnostische Beobachtungsskala für Autistische Störungen – 2

Prada P, Nicastro R, Zimmermann J, Hasler R, Aubry JM, Perroud N (2015) Addition of methylphenidate to intensive dialectical behaviour therapy for patients suffering from comorbid borderline personality disorder and ADHD: a naturalistic study. Atten Defic Hyperact Disord 7(3):199–209. doi:10.1007/s12402-015-0165-2

Roberz J, Lehmkuhl G, Sevecke K (2013) Autismus oder "Psychopathy"? Forensische Psychiatrie, Psychologie. Kriminologie 7(4):282–289

Rogers K, Dziobek I, Hassenstab J, Wolf OT, Convit A (2006) Who Cares? Revisiting empathy in Asperger syndrome. J Autism Dev Disord 37(4):709–715. doi:10.1007/s10803-006-0197-8

Rösler M, Retz W, Yaqoobi K, Burg E, Retz-Junginger P (2008) Attention deficit/hyperactivity disorder in female offenders: prevalence, psychiatric comorbidity and psychosocial implications. Eur Arch Psychiatry 259(2):98–105. doi:10.1007/s00406-008-0841-8

Scheel C, Rotarska-Jagiela A, Schilbach L, Lehnhardt FG, Krug B, Vogeley K, Tepest R (2011) Imaging derived cortical thickness reduction in high-functioning autism: key regions and temporal slope. Neuroimage 58(2):391–400. doi:10.1016/j.neuroimage.2011.06.040

Schmid M, Fegert JM, Petermann F (2010) Traumaentwicklungsstörung: Pro und Contra. Kindheit Entwicklung 19(1):47–63. doi:10.1026/0942-5403/a000008

Sevecke K, Krischer M (2008) ADHS und Persönlichkeitsstörungen bei klinisch behandelten und inhaftierten Jugendlichen. Prax Kinderpsychol Kinderpsychiatr 57:641–661

Sigman M, Dissanayake C, Corona R, Espinosa M (2003) Social and cardiac responses of young children with autism. Autism 7(2):205–216. doi:10.1177/1362361303007002007

Simonoff E, Jones CR, Baird G, Pickles A, Happe F, Charman T (2013) The persistence and stability of psychiatric problems in adolescents with autism spectrum disorders. J Child Psychol Psychiatry 54(2):186–194

Skodol AE, Gunderson JG, Shea MT, McGlashan TH, Morey LC, Sanislow CA, . . . Stout RL (2005) The Collaborative Longitudinal Personality Disorders Study (CLPS): overview and implications. J Personality Disord 19(5):487–504. doi:10.1521/pedi.2005.19.5.487

Steinhausen HC, Bisgaard C (2014) Substance use disorders in association with attention-deficit/hyperactivity disorder, co-morbid mental disorders, and medication in a nationwide sample. Eur Neuropsychopharmacol 24(2):232–241. doi:10.1016/j.euroneuro.2013.11.003

Stepp SD (2012) Development of borderline personality disorder in adolescence and young adulthood: introduction to the special section. J Abnorm Child Psychol 40(1):1–5. doi:10.1007/s10802-011-9594-3

Sucksmith E, Roth I, Hoekstra RA (2011) Autistic traits below the clinical threshold: re-examining the broader autism phenotype in the 21st century. Neuropsychol Rev 21(4):360–389

Tantam D (1988) Lifelong eccentricity and social isolation. II. Br J Psychiatry 153(6):783–791

Vannucchi G, Masi G, Toni C, Dell'Osso L, Marazziti D, Perugi G (2014) Clinical features, developmental course, and psychiatric comorbidity of adult autism spectrum disorders. CNS Spectr 19(2):157–164. doi:10.1017/s1092852913000941

Wallace GL, Dankner N, Kenworthy L, Giedd JN, Martin A (2010) Age-related temporal and parietal cortical thinning in autism spectrum disorders. Brain 133(12):3745–3754. doi:10.1093/brain/awq279

Wallace GL, Shaw P, Lee NR, Clasen LS, Raznahan A, Lenroot RK, . . . Giedd JN (2012) Distinct cortical correlates of autistic versus antisocial traits in a longitudinal sample of typically developing youth. J Neurosci 32(14):4856–4860. doi:10.1523/jneurosci.6214-11.2012

Williams K, Brignell A, Randall M, Silove N, Hazell P (2013) Selective serotonin reuptake inhibitors (SSRIs) for autism spectrum disorders (ASD). Cochrane Database Syst Rev (8):1–49. doi:10.1002/14651858.CD004677.pub3

Yang Y, Raine A, Colletti P, Toga AW, Narr KL (2009) Abnormal temporal and prefrontal cortical gray matter thinning in psychopaths. Mol Psychiatry 14(6):561–562. doi:10.1038/mp.2009.12

Young JE, Klosko JS, Weishaar M (2003) Schema therapy: a practitioner's guide. The Guilford Press, New York

"Gender Is Not on My Agenda!": Gender Dysphoria and Autism Spectrum Disorder

10

Rita George and Mark Stokes

1   Gender Dysphoria: A Disconnection Between Gender Identity and Birth Sex

Many people treat the terms "sex" and "gender" as though they were synonymous. Biological sex comprises physical attributes such as external genitalia and internal reproductive structures such as gonads, sex chromosomes, and sex hormones. Gender, on the other hand, can be a little less straightforward and is not inherently or exclusively associated to one's physical anatomy. Gender is a product of the complex interrelationship between an individual's biological sex and one's gender identity, which is an internal sense of self as male, female, both, or neither.

Most youngsters are cognizant of their gender between the ages 18 months and 3 years, and by the beginning of school years, most children will have achieved a sense of their gender identity and a certain degree of gender constancy, at which time children begin to realize that gender is a permanent state that cannot be altered by a change of clothing or activity (Paikoff and Brooks-Gunn 1991). By the age of 4 years, children typically outline preferences for the company of their same-sex peers, and by this time, boys and girls differ in interests and types of group activities and behaviors (Rosenfield and Wasserman 1993).

Gender identity can be the same or different from one's birth-assigned sex. Generally, an individual's gender identity correlates with the gender roles or attributes that a given society considers appropriate for males and females. Occasionally however, for some individuals, this is not the case. Gender dysphoria (GD) is a clinical condition where the individual experiences a persistent sense of discontentment over the incongruence between their experienced or expressed gender and their birth sex leading to significant distress to the person, an impairment of social or occupational functioning, and a desire to live a cross-gender life (Diagnostic and Statistical Manual

R. George • M. Stokes (✉)
Department of Psychology, School of Psychology, Deakin University, Geelong, Australia
e-mail: mark.stokes@deakin.edu.au

© Springer International Publishing Switzerland 2016   139
L. Mazzone, B. Vitiello (eds.), *Psychiatric Symptoms and Comorbidities in Autism Spectrum Disorder*, DOI 10.1007/978-3-319-29695-1_10

of Mental Disorders [DSM-5] (American Psychiatric Association 2013)). It is estimated that between 0.005 % and 0.014 % of natal males and 0.002–0.003 % of natal females would be diagnosed with GD, based on current diagnostic criteria (Zucker and Lawrence 2009). Expressions of GD include a preference for cross-dressing (dressing up in clothes typically worn by the opposite sex as defined by the person's cultural norms) and for stereotypical cross-gender roles and, additionally in children, make-believe play and a strong inclination for playmates of the opposite sex.

2   Gender Dysphoria (GD) and Autism Spectrum Disorder (ASD)

Interestingly, a handful of case studies (Landen and Rasmusen 1997; Tateno et al. 2008; Mukaddes 2002; Gallucci et al. 2005; Kraemer et al. 2005) attest to a comorbid presentation of ASD with GD (see Table 10.1), while empirical reports (De Vries et al. 2010; Jones et al. 2012; Pasterski et al. 2014) indicate elevated GD rates within the ASD population.

Table 10.1 Summary of case studies on the comorbid presentation of ASD and GD

Case and study	Findings
Kraemer et al. (2005) 35-year-old biological female with AS and GD	Emotionally nonreciprocating and unapproachable as a child; obstinate fascination with geometric patterns; preferred the company of male playmates, described as being tomboyish, enjoyed male stereotypical play; insisted she was a boy had an aversion to her body and secondary sex characteristics; insisted she always felt like a boy and refused girl's clothing
Galluci et al. (2005) 41-year-old biological male with AS and GD	Early developmental history remarkable for headbanging, rocking, socio-communicative impairments; preoccupation with soft fabrics, actively seeking these out; artistically talented; history of cross-dressing with women's clothing; strong desire to have the body of a woman; has fantasies of himself as a woman; expresses extreme distress with natal sex; pervasive preoccupation with physical appearance; dislikes having a penis and has confessed to wanting to use a "butcher knife to whack it off"; strongly desires sexual reassignment; obsessive need for order and predictability; passive death wish and paranoid thoughts
Tateno et al. (2008) 5-year-old male with AS and GD	The individual presented with preoccupation with colors and figures; difficulty developing peer relationships; avoided socializing; given to temper tantrums and strict adherence to own self-made rules; strong preference for female playmates; marked preoccupation with female activities abhorrence to male stereotypical toys and play; cross-dressing; disliked male body; insisted that he would grow up to be a woman; symptoms were present on follow-up for 2 years
Landen and Rasmusen (1997) 14-year-old female with AS and GD	The subject displayed echopraxia and echolalia; selective mutism; obsessive compulsions with handwashing; claimed she was a boy; refused girl's clothing or using the girl's toilet; insisted on being addressed as "he"; treatment with clomipramine helped with OCD-related symptoms but gender dysphoria persisted

Table 10.1 (continued)

Case and study	Findings
Williams et al. (1996) 5-year-old male and 3-year- and 7-month-old males with ASD and GD	Presentation included symptoms of hyperactivity, impulsivity, loneliness, and moodiness; perseverative motor activities; echolalic and echopraxic patterns; female stereotypical play and strong rejection of male pursuits; interested in Barbie dolls, related paraphernalia and female cartoon characters; ripped the heads off the dolls to play with their hair; fascinated with bright objects; preoccupation with cross-dressing, fashioned long hair from scarves; playing with dolls by shaking their hair. Described as a loner; perseverative play such as opening and closing doors; running hand repeatedly through water; prone to temper tantrums; stubbornness; favorite toys are Minnie mouse doll and Barbie doll; cross-dresses with mother's and sister's clothing and high-heeled shoes; bras and underwear; wraps shirts overhead and pretends like it is long hair
Mukaddes (2002) 10-year-old male and 7-year-old male, respectively	Subject demonstrated autistic behaviors such as restricted eye contact, unresponsiveness to verbal stimuli, echolalia, perseveration, and neologisms; developed attachment to feminine objects such as cosmetics at age 3 years; at age 6, started to cross-dress with mother's dresses, pretend to wear high heels, and express his disappointment with his gender; prayed to God to "make his penis disappear"; had fantasies about becoming a bride and being married to a man; complete disinterest in rough-tumble play typical of males; preferred the company of girls
	Subject presented with a history of delayed language; difficulties with social-affective development and eye contact; stereotypical behaviors, toe walking, and a low frustration tolerance; at the age of 4–5 years started some make-believe play, such as "playing house" and "playing mother roles"; avoided rough-tumble male-oriented play and preferred the company of his mother and female classmates; persistently expressed his desire to grow up to be a woman like his mother and enjoyed making skirts with his mother's scarves
Perera et al. (2003) 20-year-old female with AS, GD, and OCD	The case presented with socially awkward behavior; rejection of all peer-group activities; classroom disruptive behavior; indiscriminate and frequent aggression; recurrent compulsion; parents distressed about her strange obsession with licking public floors; confession to irrational compulsive fears about parents dying; high achiever in school and artistically talented; at age of 14 years, started to experience gender-dysphoric symptoms; voiced deep resentment to her gender and insisted on being a male; physically violent to those who resisted her thinking insisted on sexual reassignment surgery and hormonal treatments after menarche; patient was diagnosed with OCD and AS; medication with clomipramine alleviated some of the OCD symptoms, with less overt GD symptoms

When using the Diagnostic Interview for Social and Communication Disorders (Leekam et al. 2002), a group of Dutch researchers found an incidence of 7.8 % of ASD among a sample of children and adolescents referred to a gender identity clinic for management of their GD ($N = 204$, $Mage = 10.8$ years, $SD = 3.58$). This rate is much higher than the prevalence rate of ASD in the general population which ranges from 0.6 % to 2 % (Fombonne 2005; Blumberg et al. 2013). Similarly, employing the Autism Spectrum Quotient (AQ, Baron-Cohen et al. 2003), a standardized test to measure autistic characteristics, Jones et al. (2012) demonstrated that 14.8% of female adults with GD ($N=61$) and 3% of male adults with GD ($N=198$) met the criteria for a potential diagnosis of ASD, while Pasterski et al. (2014) also testified to the ASD-GD association among adults in their sample, where 7.1% of the females with GD ($N=28$) and 4.7% of males with GD ($N=63$) met diagnostic criteria according to the recommended cutoff scores on the AQ.

While some research has assessed for ASD traits in a population referred for GD, newer research by Strang et al. (2014) measured gender variance, defined as the desire to be the opposite gender, in a population of children with ASD ($N=147$). On analyzing parental responses to the item "Wishes to be the opposite sex" on the Child Behavior Checklist (CBCL), gender variance was 7.59 times higher in the ASD group than in the non-ASD participants, which comprised of a community sample ($N=165$) and normative data from the non-referred standardization sample of the CBCL ($N=1,605$). Bejerot and Eriksson (2014) similarly demonstrated a gender-atypical pattern (males were less masculine and females were less feminine) in their sample of 50 adults with ASD when compared to 53 typically developing individuals.

George and Stokes (submitted) measured gender-dysphoric symptomology in an international population of adults diagnosed with ASD ($N=220$), using a mixed methods approach. In their quantitative study, using the Gender Dysphoria and Gender Identity Questionnaire (GIDQ-AA, Deogracias et al. 2007), results demonstrated that individuals with ASD were significantly more likely to report experiencing gender-dysphoric symptoms than were typically developing individuals (Cohen's $d=0.63$). In a subsequent qualitative analysis investigating gender-related attitudes among 94 adults with ASD, female participants reported that it was easier to identify with males and that they were not like other women in that "vulnerability, nurturing and intimacy is not natural to me" and that men were more "straightforward, easier to understand," "blunt," and "did not bother with emotional stuff." Male participants also conceded to feeling "sensitive, shy and introverted," "not fitting the typical male stereotype," and not enjoying sports and "stereotypical male socializing activities" but divulged that their disconnection from other men was not primarily due to gender issues, but due to ASD-related issues. Taken together, an androgynous self-concept, gender ambivalence, and dissatisfaction with culturally dictated gender roles emerged as dominant themes in the discourse.

3   Why Would Gender Dysphoria Be More Prevalent in ASD?

3.1   Hormonal Factors and GD

The coexistence of ASD and GD is worth noting as the prevalence of both conditions is reasonably low. Reasons for this comorbidity have been a topic of emerging interest, and several plausible speculations have been proposed to account for this association. Some researchers have hypothesized that perhaps ASD is the driver that predisposes some individuals to GD (Kraemer et al. 2005). A neurobiological mechanism might provide some explanation. The "extreme male brain" theory of ASD (Baron-Cohen 2002) argues that fetal testosterone or fT is a strong candidate for contributing to sexually dimorphic cognition and behavior and may present a risk factor for conditions characterized by social impairments, such as ASD (Knickmeyer and Baron-Cohen 2006), where individuals with ASD may demonstrate characteristics generally associated with masculinity, such as an overdevelopment of logical thinking, low emotionality, and high level of perseverance. Elevated levels of fT are positively correlated with autistic traits and with masculinizing neural development (Auyeung et al. 2009). The hypothesis that fT levels influence human sexual behavior derives from a large body of research on the neural and behavioral effects of early hormone manipulations among rodents and nonhuman primates (Hines et al. 2004). Castrated males show feminized cognition and behaviors, while conversely females treated with testosterone show corresponding masculinization (Knickmeyer et al. 2005; Berenbaum et al. 2009).

Information on the influence of fT on neural and behavior development in humans may be derived from clinical literature where the amount or activity of fT is disrupted, such as among women with congenital adrenal hyperplasia (CAH) and men with complete androgen insensitivity syndrome (CAIS). The prenatal exposure to unusually high levels of fT among girls with CAH is hypothesized to influence sexual development. Girls with CAH show increased male-typical play behaviors (Hines et al. 2004), masculinized gender identities (Dessens et al. 2005), and homosexual and bisexual orientations (Meyer-Bahlburg et al. 2008). Interestingly, an increased number of autistic traits as measured on the AQ were also noted in this group (Knickmeyer et al. 2006). The opposite pattern of a female-typical psychosexual development is demonstrated by men with CAIS, an X-linked disorder characterized by a complete absence of functional androgen receptors (Hines et al. 2004). These pathways provide an explanation for GD among females with ASD; the predisposing dual role of elevated levels of fT in ASD and in male gender identity development (Gooren 2006) points to one possible neurohormonal explanatory pathway for the co-occurrence of GD and ASD among females, where a primarily masculine cognition and self-perception in ASD may be lead females with ASD to interpret themselves as masculine relative to their same-sex peers, and this then could pave the way to the development of GD.

However, when viewed through the same theoretical lens, elevated fT levels do not provide a very forthright explanation for increased rates of GD among males within ASD. Higher levels of fT would be expected to hypermasculinize the male brain and thus allow for a pronounced male gender identity. Given the association between elevated levels of fT in ASD, why then would males with ASD demonstrate higher rates of GD, when the converse would be expected or, at the least, similar rates of GD among ASD and TD males?

MacCulloch and Waddington (1981) and Pillard and Weinrich (1987) have suggested that human sexual orientation depends on, among other factors, differences in the degree of in utero masculinization and behavioral defeminization of the brain, where the "default brain" is believed to be female. Support for such a model comes from observations on gender-dependent cognitive abilities that are mostly female-like in homosexual males (Robinson and Manning 2000). Research into the existence of neuroendocrinological differences between homosexual and heterosexual men may be reflective of a partially female-differentiated neural circuitry in homosexual males (Dorner et al. 1975; Gladue et al. 1984). While this finding has prompted the assumption that homosexual males have been exposed to low levels of fT, a number of researchers have challenged this idea (McFadden and Champlin 2000; Rahman and Wilson 2003; Williams et al. 2000; Jenkins 2010). Studies looking into somatic features such as finger length ratios (Robinson and Manning 2000) and male genitalia proportions (Bogaert and Hershberger 1999) tend to support the conclusion that elevated levels of prenatal testosterone might predispose the male fetus to homosexuality.

More recent literature has found a relationship between another sexually dimorphic sex hormone, the anti-Müllerian hormone (AMH), and ASD, where lower levels of AMH have been associated with increased ASD symptoms in males (Pankhurst and McLennan 2012). AMH is believed to play a role in the masculinization of or the defeminization of the male fetus (Behringer et al. 1994), and whether lower levels of AMH contribute in any way to a less masculinized brain, which could then lend itself to a higher risk for gender dysphoria, has not yet been researched, but provides a promising avenue for future research.

Given the shared pathways between elevated fT and ASD, elevated fT and male homosexuality, the predilection for a higher rate of female-type cognition, and behaviors among male homosexuals, together with the higher prevalence rates of male homosexuality in ASD (George and Stokes submitted), perhaps the correlations between the different variables in this biological model could provide one possible instructive pathway for the high rates of GD among ASD males.

To limit a construct as complex as gender identity to biological factors would be overly reductionistic. While there is no consensus in the scientific community on why a person develops a particular gender identity (American Psychological Association, 2013), an individual's gender identity would most likely be an interaction of their physiology with their social environment. Specifically, certain features characteristic to ASD may increase the risk for GD (VanderLaan et al. 2015).

3.2   ASD-Specific Features and GD

The general consensus among researchers looking into the ASD-GD association was that "autistic-like" traits were possibly driving GD. It is speculated that sensory issues characteristic of ASD may hinder what is perceived as normative gendered behavior. Categorizing individuals into a binary gender system on the conjecture of clothing may not be of much relevance to many individuals with ASD, where the primary focus may sometimes be on a preference for specific sensory input, featural details, or tactile sensation (Tateno et al. 2008; de Vries et al. 2010) and not social norms. Consistently, in George and Stokes's (submitted) study, male responses indicated that they preferred softer, glittery, and silkier fabrics, not because they were "girly" clothes, but because "of my autism." Female responses similarly suggested that "girly clothes were tight and itchy," "makeup felt terrible," and "men's clothes were comfortable, straightforward, and practical."

Communication difficulties are characteristic of ASD, and some individuals with ASD may have challenges recognizing gender due to linguistics. Since gender relies on semantic factors (Eckert and McConnell-Ginet 2003; Labov 2011), language delays during childhood may also interfere with a developing sense of gender-related discourse, where, without words for "boy-girl," "pink-blue," or "trucks-dolls," for example, or without employing these words in appropriate contexts, one may not develop a clear understanding of gendered behavior.

It has been suggested that another ASD-specific feature that may play a role in the ASD-GD association is the frequent presence of obsessive compulsive behaviors in ASD (Gallucci et al. 2005). The DSM-5 includes intense/obsessional interests and repetitive behaviors as part of the diagnostic criteria for ASD, and pharmacological studies have created a compelling argument for the association between ASD and obsessive compulsive disorder (Hollander et al. 2006). Thus, a rather intriguing speculation is that in some individuals with ASD, GD may develop as a sequel to ASD, where one's unusual preoccupations with cross-gender activities and objects may not be related to gender identity confusion in the truest sense, but may just be part of the symptomology of ASD. Findings reported by the VanderLaan et al. (2015) study are consistent with this argument. They found that a sample of 534 children clinically referred for GD showed an elevation in intense and obsessional interests on responses to an item on the CBCL which measures obsessions and compulsions, when compared to CBCL clinic-referred and non-referred standardization samples. The pervasive preoccupations and distress with cross-gender roles, restricted related interests, and sometimes ritualized behavior seen in clients with GD could be one manifestation of obsessive behaviors inherent to ASD, and other researchers have agreed to this (Landén and Rasmussen 1997; Perera and Gadambanathan 2003; Gallucci et al. 2005).

3.3   Gender Is Socio-Rhetorical

Gender identity typically forms around 3–4 years of age and is considered a social developmental marker (Robinow 2009). Literature has reliably demonstrated that early positive social interactions are critical to the development of a fund of higher-order social skills (Parker and Asher 1993), which in turn is pivotal to the development and healthy expression of gender and sexuality (Gagnon and Simon 2011; Rees et al. 2006). Given that impaired social functioning is a hallmark feature of ASD, the establishment of a gender identity could become complex. Additionally, drawing on the theory of mind in relation to autism, deficits with empathy and imagination may further hinder the development of a view of oneself as belonging to a gender group (Happé and Frith 1995).

Abelson (1981) indicated that the establishment of gender identity in children with autism appeared to be a function of their social communication. He went on to stress that achieving gender identity is a critical milestone for children as this would then go on to facilitate forming effective emotional bonds with their identified gender group, which would then help forge meaningful and appropriate social relationships. A rather vicious circle is speculated here, where deficiencies in their social skills raise challenges for the child with ASD to come to a clear understanding of their gender identity, and then a fragmented or dysfunctional gender identity interferes with the child's integration into their own gender group, placing them at a disadvantage to develop healthy social bonds with their peers. However, it must be stressed that, clearly, not all children with ASD struggle with their gender identity and many go on to have a clear understanding of their gender (Abelson 1981).

Accordingly, on investigating attitudes of individuals with ASD to gender identity, George and Stokes (submitted) found that 83 % of the responses from males and 94 % of responses from females indicated that gender was conceptualized as a socio-rhetorical system. Participants shared that the system was not always straightforward to negotiate for the individual with ASD and that gender would best be described as "fluid, a socially restrictive label, confusing, outdated, and irrelevant to their personal identity." Furthermore, many participants shared sentiments on being more content with a "genderless society." Other authors diagnosed with ASD shared similar sentiments and confessed that their "nervous system is configured differently" (Golubock 2003) and that their wiring just would not "understand, interpret, and perform gender-typing" effortlessly and without conflict and conceded to "gender-blindness" (Meyerding 2003). Perhaps then, examining gender from the perspective of someone with ASD licenses a denaturalization of social norms and expectations.

4   Management of GD

While for many individuals with ASD, a gender-fluid lifestyle may not hinder social, mental, and occupational functioning, for some the incongruence between their perceived gender identity and their birth sex could develop into a GD, as was evident in the increased number of ASD diagnoses among clients referred to gender clinics for clinical management (Jones et al. 2012; Pasterski et al. 2014). This is understandable, given that the rigid thinking styles characteristic of ASD would not lend itself to a dissonance between one's thoughts and their behavior. George and Stokes (submitted) similarly found significantly higher scores on their GD survey among ASD participants; three individuals scored over the cutoff point, warranting a diagnosis of GD. This rate of 1.4 % was much higher than found in the general population, approximately 560 times higher than the prevalence rates in the wider population.

Living with GD can be extremely distressing to the individual, and treatment is generally aimed at alleviating this distress by helping the individuals with GD live their lives the way they would like to, in their preferred gender identity. What this means would vary from person to person and thus management of GD is undertaken on a case to case basis. For individuals under the age of 18 years of age, a multidisciplinary team, comprising specialists from the mental health profession and pediatric endocrinologists, is called upon to provide assistance to the child and the family. For children under the age of 12, support provided is mostly psychological, rather than medical or surgical. This is because in most gender-dysphoric children, GD will cease when they reach puberty (Wallien and Cohen-Kettenis 2008). Psychological support offers children and their families a chance to discuss their thoughts and receive support to help them emotionally cope with their distress, without rushing into more drastic treatments.

However, if GD persists into adolescence, hormonal treatment is commenced sometimes with gonadotropin-releasing hormone (GnRH) analogs, which suppress pubertal hormones responsible for bringing about physical changes to the body related to one's biological sex (Hembree et al. 2009). GnRH can aid with the delay of these potentially distressing physical changes until the individual with GD is old enough for more radical treatment options. Treatment with GnRH is reversible and gives the young person time to consider their choices and make informed decisions regarding their future course.

Once the young person reaches the age of 18, management will be transferred to gender identity clinics that specialize in support and treatment of adults with GD (Hembree et al. 2008). At this stage, both the individual and the medical team are more confident in their course of action, and permanent pharmacological treatment such as masculinizing or feminizing hormones and surgical treatment through sexual reassignment are available to alter the individual's physical appearance to further line up with their gender identity.

However, when an individual with GD presents with co-occurring ASD, the level of complexity in terms of clinical management increases, owing to the comorbid presence of symptoms of both GD and ASD. In treating the GD, the ASD will need to be taken into account, and disentangling whether the GD is indeed a separate condition and not related to ASD-related symptoms remains a challenge to provide individuals with comorbid ASD and GD with proper care (De Vries et al. 2010). Having a diagnosis of ASD need not affect whether the individual continues on their chosen path for sexual reassignment surgery but, considering the diagnosis, may assist the individual in examining the motives behind their choices and accordingly make better informed decisions about treatment and physical mediations.

Conclusions

Possibly the most fundamental characteristic of a person's identity is their gender, which conceivably deeply influences every part of one's life. In a society where this crucial aspect of self has been so narrowly defined and rigidly enforced, individuals who exist outside its norms likely face innumerable challenges and can become targets of disapproval. An individual diagnosed with ASD and experiencing GD would understandably bear a significant burden of distress, and George and Stokes (submitted) found levels of depression, anxiety, and stress positively correlated with the levels of GD symptomology reported by individuals with ASD.

Gender is possibly the one most intensively socialized construct, with many "rules" that are not explicit, and while these gendered norms are typically reflexively embodied by most persons, it is reasonable that gender may be somewhat challenging for some individuals with ASD. The confusion of navigating within this milieu may manifest as GD in some cases of individuals with ASD, when it might be an ASD identity versus a neurotypical identity that may be at the core of their identity issue, rather than a clear desire for a cross-gendered lifestyle. Indeed, this tension could contribute to the development of a true GD. Equally tenable is the possibility that ASD may share a common pathway with the pathophysiology of GD, an avenue that requires careful empirical clarification.

GD is overrepresented in ASD when compared to the general population. While we cannot say with any certainty that gender identity is impervious to biological influences or that gender identity is free of social influences, we suggest that the relative balance of biological and social influences may be more variant and synergistic, on average, for individuals with ASD than for TD individuals.

References

Abelson AG (1981) The development of gender identity in the autistic child. Child Care Health Dev 7(6):347–356

American Psychiatric Association (2013) Diagnostic and statistical manual of mental disorders (5th ed.).

Auyeung B, Baron-Cohen S, Ashwin E, Knickmeyer R, Taylor K, Hackett G (2009) Fetal testosterone and autistic traits. Br J Psychol 100(1):1–22

Baron-Cohen S (2002) The extreme male brain theory of autism. Trends Cogn Sci 6(6):248–254

Baron-Cohen S, Richler J, Bisarya D, Gurunathan N, Wheelwright S (2003) The systemizing quotient: an investigation of adults with Asperger syndrome or high–functioning autism, and normal sex differences. Philos Trans R Soc Lond B: Biol Sci 358(1430):361–374

Behringer RR, Finegold MJ, Cate RL (1994) Müllerian-inhibiting substance function during mammalian sexual development. Cell 79(3):415–425

Bejerot S, Eriksson JM (2014) Sexuality and gender role in autism spectrum disorder: a case control study. PLoS One 9(1):e87961

Berenbaum SA, Bryk KK, Nowak N, Quigley CA, Moffat S (2009) Fingers as a marker of prenatal androgen exposure. Endocrinology 150(11):5119–5124

Blumberg SJ, Bramlett MD, Kogan MD, Schieve LA, Jones JR, Lu MC (2013) Changes in prevalence of parent-reported autism spectrum disorder in school-aged US children: 2007 to 2011–2012. Natl Health Stat Rep 65(20):1–7

Bogaert AF, Hershberger S (1999) The relation between sexual orientation and penile size. Arch Sex Behav 28(3):213–221

De Vries AL, Noens IL, Cohen-Kettenis PT, van Berckelaer-Onnes IA, Doreleijers TA (2010) Autism spectrum disorders in gender dysphoric children and adolescents. J Autism Dev Disord 40(8):930–936

Deogracias JJ, Johnson LL, Meyer-Bahlburg HF, Kessler SJ, Schober JM, Zucker KJ (2007) The gender identity/gender dysphoria questionnaire for adolescents and adults. J Sex Res 44(4):370–379

Dessens AB, Slijper FM, Drop SL (2005) Gender dysphoria and gender change in chromosomal females with congenital adrenal hyperplasia. Arch Sex Behav 34(4):389–397

Dörner G, Rohde W, Stahl F, Krell L, Masius WG (1975) A neuroendocrine predisposition for homosexuality in men. Arch Sex Behav 4(1):1–8

Eckert P, McConnell-Ginet S (2003) Language and gender. Cambridge University Press

Fombonne E (2005) The changing epidemiology of autism. J Appl Res Intellect Disabil 18(4):281–294

Gagnon JH, Simon W (2011) *Sexual conduct: The social sources of human sexuality*. Transaction Publishers, Piscataway

Gallucci G, Hackerman F, Schmidt CW Jr (2005) Gender identity disorder in an adult male with Asperger's syndrome. Sex Disabil 23(1):35–40

George R, Stokes MA (submitted) Sexual orientation and gender-identity among high functioning individuals with autism spectrum disorder

Gladue BA, Green R, Hellman RE (1984) Neuroendocrine response to estrogen and sexual orientation. Science 225(4669):1496–1499

Golubock S (2003) Different on the inside. In: Miller JK (ed) Women from another planet? Our lives in the universe of autism. 1st Books Library, Fairfield, pp 157–70, Print

Gooren L (2006) The biology of human psychosexual differentiation. Horm Behav 50(4):589–601

Happé F, Frith U (1995) Theory of mind in autism. In: Learning and cognition in autism. Springer US, pp 177–97

Hembree WC, Cohen-Kettenis P, Delemarre-van de Waal HA, Gooren LJ, Meyer III WJ, Spack NP, Tangpricha V, Montori VM (2009) Endocrine treatment of transsexual persons: an Endocrine Society clinical practice guideline. *J Clin Endocrinol Metab* 94(9): 3132–3154

Hines M, Brook C, Conway GS (2004) Androgen and psychosexual development: core gender identity, sexual orientation, and recalled childhood gender role behavior in women and men with congenital adrenal hyperplasia (CAH). J Sex Res 41(1):75–81

Hollander E, Soorya L, Wasserman S, Esposito K, Chaplin W, Anagnostou E (2006) Divalproex sodium vs. placebo in the treatment of repetitive behaviours in autism spectrum disorder. Int J Neuropsychopharmacol 9(02):209–213

Jenkins WJ (2010) Can anyone tell me why I'm gay? What research suggests regarding the origins of sexual orientation. N Am J Psychol 12(2):279

Jones RM, Wheelwright S, Farrell K, Martin E, Green R, Di Ceglie D, Baron-Cohen S (2012) Brief report: female-to-male transsexual people and autistic traits. J Autism Dev Disord 42(2):301–306

Knickmeyer RC, Baron-Cohen S (2006) Topical review: fetal testosterone and sex differences in typical social development and in autism. J Child Neurol 21(10):825–845

Knickmeyer RC, Wheelwright S, Taylor K, Raggatt P, Hackett G, Baron-Cohen S (2005) Gender-typed play and amniotic testosterone. Dev Psychol 41(3):517

Knickmeyer R, Baron-Cohen S, Fane BA, Wheelwright S, Mathews GA, Conway GS, Brook CG, Hines M (2006) Androgens and autistic traits: A study of individuals with congenital adrenal hyperplasia. Horm Behav 50(1):148–53. Epub 2006 Apr 19

Kraemer B, Delsignore A, Gundelfinger R, Schnyder U, Hepp U (2005) Comorbidity of Asperger syndrome and gender identity disorder. Eur Child Adolesc Psychiatry 14(5):292–296

Labov W (2011) *Principles of linguistic change, cognitive and cultural factors*, (Vol. 3). John Wiley & Sons

Landén M, Rasmussen P (1997) Gender identity disorder in a girl with autism—a case report. Eur Child Adolesc Psychiatry 6(3):170–173

Leekam SR, Libby SJ, Wing L, Gould J, Taylor C (2002) The diagnostic interview for social and communication disorders: algorithms for ICD-10 childhood autism and wing and Gould autistic spectrum disorder. J Child Psychol Psychiatry 43(3):327–342

MacCulloch MJ, Waddington JL (1981) Neuroendocrine mechanisms and the aetiology of male and female homosexuality. Br J Psychiatry 139(4):341–345

McFadden D, Champlin CA (2000) Comparison of auditory evoked potentials in heterosexual, homosexual, and bisexual males and females. J Assoc Res Otolaryngol 1(1):89–99

Meyer-Bahlburg HF, Dolezal C, Baker SW, New MI (2008) Sexual orientation in women with classical or non-classical congenital adrenal hyperplasia as a function of degree of prenatal androgen excess. Arch Sex Behav 37(1):85–99

Meyerding J (2003) Growing up genderless. In: Miller JK (ed) Women from another planet? Our lives in the universe of autism. 1st Books Library, Fairfield, pp 157–70, Print

Mukaddes NM (2002) Gender identity problems in autistic children. Child Care Health Dev 28(6):529–532

Paikoff RL, Brooks-Gunn J (1991) Do parent-child relationships change during puberty? Psychol Bull 110(1):47

Pankhurst MW, McLennan IS (2012) Inhibin B and anti-Müllerian hormone/Müllerian-inhibiting substance may contribute to the male bias in autism. Transl Psychiatry 2(8):e148

Parker JG, Asher SR (1993) Friendship and friendship quality in middle childhood: links with peer group acceptance and feelings of loneliness and social dissatisfaction. Dev Psychol 29(4):611

Pasterski V, Gilligan L, Curtis R (2014) Traits of autism spectrum disorders in adults with gender dysphoria. *Arch Sex Behav*, 43(2):387–393

Perera H, Gadambanathan T, Weerasiri S (2003) Gender identity disorder presenting in a girl with Asperger's disorder and obsessive compulsive disorder. Ceylon Med J 48(2):57–58

Pillard RC, Weinrich JD (1987) The periodic table model of the gender transpositions: part I. A theory based on masculinization and defeminization of the brain. J Sex Res 23(4):425–454

Rahman Q, Wilson GD (2003) Sexual orientation and the 2nd to 4th finger length ratio: evidence for organising effects of sex hormones or developmental instability? Psychoneuroendocrinology 28(3):288–303

Rees AM, Doyle C, Miesch J. Sexual orientation, gender role expression, and stereotyping: the intersection between sexism and sexual prejudice (homophobia). Vistas 2006 Online

Robinow O (2009) Paraphilia and transgenderism: a connection with Asperger's disorder? Sex Relatsh Ther 24(2):143–151

Robinson SJ, Manning JT (2000) The ratio of 2nd to 4th digit length and male homosexuality. Evol Hum Behav 21(5):333–345

Rosenfield A, Wasserman S (1993) Sexual development in the early school-aged child. Child Adolesc Psychiatr Clin N Am 2:393–406

Strang JF, Kenworthy L, Dominska A, Sokoloff J, Kenealy LE, Berl M, … Wallace GL (2014) Increased gender variance in autism spectrum disorders and attention deficit hyperactivity disorder. Arch Sex Behav 43(8):1525–1533

Tateno M, Tateno Y, Saito T (2008) Comorbid childhood gender identity disorder in a boy with Asperger syndrome. Psychiatry Clin Neurosci 62(2):238–238

VanderLaan DP, Postema L, Wood H, Singh D, Fantus S, Hyun J, … Zucker KJ (2015) Do children with gender dysphoria have intense/obsessional interests?. J Sex R 52(2):213–219

Wallien MS, Cohen-Kettenis PT (2008) Psychosexual outcome of gender-dysphoric children. J Am Acad Child Adolesc Psychiatry 47(12):1413–1423

Williams PG, Allard AM, Sears L (1996) Case study: cross-gender preoccupations with two male children with autism. J Autism Dev Disord 26(6):635–642

Williams TJ, Pepitone ME, Christensen SE, Cooke BM, Huberman AD, Breedlove NJ, … Breedlove SM (2000) Finger-length ratios and sexual orientation. Nature 404(6777):455–456

Zucker KJ, Lawrence AA (2009) Epidemiology of gender identity disorder: recommendations for the standards of care of the world professional association for transgender health. Int J Transgenderism 11(1):8–18

Index

© Springer International Publishing Switzerland 2016   151
L. Mazzone, B. Vitiello (eds.), *Psychiatric Symptoms and Comorbidities in
Autism Spectrum Disorder*, DOI 10.1007/978-3-319-29695-1

Printed by Printforce, the Netherlands